Contents

Home and Leisure Injuries in the United States

A Compendium of Articles from the
Morbidity and Mortality Weekly Report, 1985-1995

Compiled by

Judy A. Stevens, MS, MPH
Christine M. Branche-Dorsey, PhD

National Center for Injury Prevention and Control
Atlanta, Georgia
1996

This compendium is a publication of the National Center for Injury
Prevention and Control of the Centers for Disease Control and Prevention:

Centers for Disease Control and Prevention
David Satcher, MD, PhD, Director

National Center for Injury Prevention and Control
Mark L. Rosenberg, MD, MPP, Director

Division of Unintentional Injury Prevention
David A. Sleet, PhD, Acting Director

Home and Leisure Injury Prevention Team
Christine M. Branche-Dorsey, PhD, Leader

Production services were provided by the staff of the Office of Health
Communications, National Center for Injury Prevention and Control:

Technical Information Services
Sandra E. Bonzo

Editing
Valerie R. Johnson

Cover Design
Mary Ann Braun

Layout
Sandra S. Emrich

Suggested Citation: National Center for Injury Prevention and Control.
Home and leisure injuries in the United States: a compendium of articles
from the Morbidity and Mortality Weekly Report, 1985–1995. Atlanta,
GA: Centers for Disease Control and Prevention, 1996.

Introduction

Injury prevention is a major public health issue. Home and leisure injuries occur during everyday activities and affect people of all ages, socioeconomic levels, and occupations. The scope of this report includes falls, fires and burns, drownings, injuries due to sports and leisure activities, and poisonings. Each year, these types of injuries account for nearly 700,000 deaths and millions of nonfatal injuries. In 1992, falls, fire and burn injuries, drownings, and poisonings were responsible for 28,717 deaths. Injuries are the leading cause of hospital admissions for persons under 45 years of age. Nonfatal injuries result in 114 million physician contacts each year, and more than 25% of all emergency department or hospital clinic visits are for treatment of injuries. Injuries incur a huge economic burden; current financial costs from injuries are estimated at $224 billion per year.

As part of its prevention activities, the Division of Unintentional Injury Prevention (DUIP) in the Centers for Disease Control and Prevention's National Center for Injury Prevention and Control (NCIPC) conducts and coordinates scientific activities through intramural and extramural research, surveillance, and programs at the state, local, and community levels. In collaboration with state and local health departments, other federal agencies, private partners, and community-based organizations, DUIP has published research findings in the *Morbidity and Mortality Weekly Report* (*MMWR*) describing the extent and impact of a variety of home and leisure injury problems and has provided suggestions for reducing these injuries by applying public health interventions and prevention strategies.

This compendium contains all of the *MMWR* articles concerning home and leisure injuries published from 1985 through 1995; a summary public health message precedes each article. The articles cover a wide variety of topics, ranging from hunting injuries to poisonings. The public health approach to preventing home and leisure injuries represented in this compilation covers areas related to surveillance, risk factors, and interventions. We have organized this compendium of *MMWR* articles by the following subject areas:

- unintentional injuries and surveillance
- economic impact
- falls
- fires and burns
- sports and leisure activities
- poisonings

Strategies to reduce home and leisure injuries include a focus on technology and engineering solutions, education and behavior changes, and legislation and law enforcement. No single approach is likely to produce as much benefit as applying a combination of strategies simultaneously. Accordingly, these *MMWR* articles focus on approaches that apply relevant combinations of strategies to a range of home and leisure injury problems.

Injury control professionals face new challenges in the coming decade, including identifying new populations at risk for injuries and developing and testing programs that are innovative and effective in preventing injuries. Achieving these goals will require the collaboration of physicians, health care providers, and state and local health departments and agencies as well as parents, consumer groups, teachers, product manufacturers, law enforcement personnel, social service and housing agencies, city planners, and other community members interested in injury control and public health.

Unintentional Injuries and Surveillance

Fatal Injuries to Children — United States, 1986

Effective interventions for reducing childhood fatalities in the home are the installation of swimming pool enclosures, the use of smoke detectors, and the use of antiscald devices in showerheads and faucets.

—MMWR Vol. 39/No. 26, July 6, 1990, pp. 442–5, 451

Fatal Injuries to Children — United States, 1986

Injuries are a leading cause of mortality among children ≤19 years of age in the United States (1). As part of the Injury Prevention Act of 1986,* Congress requested that the Secretary of Health and Human Services, through CDC, analyze the causes and incidence of childhood injuries in the United States and make recommendations for injury prevention and control legislation. The Secretary's report, *Childhood Injuries in the United States: A Report to Congress* (2), was presented to Congress in October 1989; it was based on national data for 1986 maintained by CDC's National Center for Health Statistics and on research conducted by pediatric injury experts in the United States. This report summarizes mortality data from *Childhood Injuries in the United States* for children (defined as persons aged ≤19 years) from the five leading causes of fatal injuries to children in the United States in 1986 (i.e., motor vehicle crashes, homicide, suicide, drowning, and fires/burns).

Motor Vehicle Crashes

Motor vehicle crashes accounted for almost half of the 22,411 fatal injuries among children in the United States (Table 1); a substantial proportion (an estimated 15%–30%) of these deaths were associated with alcohol use (3). Of all motor vehicle-related fatalities, 70% occurred among motor vehicle occupants, and 17%, among pedestrians. Occupant fatality rates for 15–19-year-olds (30.7 per 100,000) from motor vehicle crashes were 10 times those for children <10 years of age (3.0 per 100,000).

Among children aged 5–9 years, pedestrian injuries were associated with more deaths (502 [24%] of 2133) than any other cause of injury. Regardless of race, fatality rates for male pedestrians ≤19 years of age (3.2 per 100,000) were nearly twice as high as those for females (1.8 per 100.000); rates for children of races other than white (3.5 per 100,000) were 1.5 times those for white children (2.3 per 100,000).

TABLE 1. Number, percentage, and rate of fatal injuries for children ≤19 years of age, by leading cause of injury — United States, 1986

Cause of injury	No.	(%)	Rate per 100,000
Motor vehicle crash	10,535	(47.0)	14.9
Occupant	7,412	(33.0)	10.5
Pedestrian	1,787	(8.0)	2.5
Other	1,336	(6.0)	1.9
Homicide	2,877	(12.8)	4.1
Suicide	2,151	(9.6)	3.0
Drowning	2,062	(9.2)	2.9
Fire/Burns	1,619	(7.2)	2.3
Other	3,167	(14.1)	4.5
All	**22,411**	**(100.0)**	**31.7**

---

*Public Law no. 99-649, § 1, 100 Stat. 3633 (42 U.S.C. § 201 [1989]).

Homicide

In 1986, deaths due to homicide accounted for nearly 13% of fatal injuries among children (Table 1). Nearly two thirds of childhood homicide deaths were among 15–19-year-olds; however, 23% were among children <5 years of age. Sixty-eight percent of homicide deaths were among males. Rates for black children (12.2 per 100,000) were approximately five times those for white children (2.6 per 100,000). Sixty-one percent of homicides among males and 32% of homicides among females involved firearms.

Suicide

Suicide was the third leading cause of childhood fatal injuries (Table 1). Among 10–19-year-olds, males accounted for 80% of suicides; of these, an estimated 60% were associated with firearms. Age-specific rates among white children were generally 1.5–2.5 times the suicide rate for black children.

Drowning

Drowning, the fourth leading cause of childhood fatal injuries, was most common among children ≤4 years of age and males aged 15–19 years. Among the latter group, drownings occurred in a wide variety of aquatic environments; alcohol use was associated with an estimated 40%–50% of these events. Drowning rates for black children (4.5 per 100,000) were almost twice those for white children (2.6 per 100,000). In three states (Arizona, California, and Florida), drowning was the leading cause of fatal injuries for children ≤4 years of age. In all states, up to 90% of drownings among this age group occurred in residential swimming pools.

Fire/Burns

Fire/burns were the fifth leading cause of childhood death from injury. Fifty-three percent of childhood burn deaths occurred among children aged ≤4 years and 73% among children ≤9 years of age. Fire/burn deaths were more common among black children (5.1 per 100,000) than among children of other races (1.8 per 100,000). For children ≤9 years of age, black males (8.4 per 100,000) were three times more likely than white males (2.8 per 100,000) and black females (8.6 per 100,000) 4.5 times more likely than white females (2.0 per 100,000) to die in a house fire. Overall, 80% of deaths from fire/burns resulted from house fires, 9% from electrical burns, and 2% from scalding.

Reported by: Div of Injury Control, Center for Environmental Health and Injury Control, CDC.

Editorial Note: *Childhood Injuries in the United States: A Report to Congress* (2) provides the first comprehensive assessment of childhood injuries in the United States and underscores how the relative importance of childhood injuries has increased over the last 20 years. From 1968 through 1986, death rates for children from noninjury causes have declined 56%, while death rates from injuries have declined 22% (Figure 1). Injuries are the leading cause of death among children and account for as many years of potential life lost before age 65 as the next two leading categories—congenital anomalies and prematurity—combined (Figure 2).

Each year, injuries account for 20% of all hospitalizations among U.S. children, nearly 16 million emergency room visits, and permanent disability to more than 30,000 children (4). Although the direct and indirect costs of these injuries are difficult to measure, in 1982, the estimated costs exceeded $7.5 billion (5); in 1985, they were nearly $8.3 billion, with lifetime costs exceeding $13 billion (6).

FIGURE 1. Death rates* for children ≤19 years of age from injuries and other diseases — United States, 1968–1986

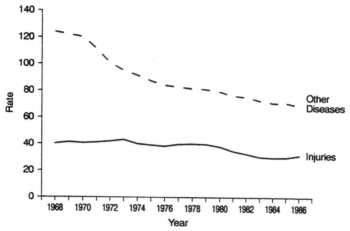

*Per 100,000 population.

FIGURE 2. Years of potential life lost (YPLL) before age 65 among children ≤19 years of age from injuries and other diseases — United States, 1986

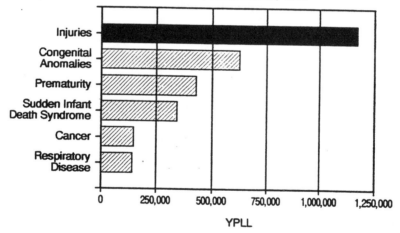

For many childhood injuries, effective interventions are being developed or already exist and have been implemented. For example, morbidity and/or mortality from injuries could be reduced for 1) motor vehicle crashes by air bags, automatic occupant restraints, antilock brakes, programs to reduce drug and alcohol abuse, and barriers to separate pedestrians from traffic; 2) homicide by teaching conflict resolution skills and by reduction of access to lethal weapons such as firearms (7);

3) suicide by improved identification and referral of persons at high risk for suicide and efforts to limit access to lethal means of suicide such as firearms, high places, and prescription drugs (7,8); 4) drowning by enclosure of swimming pools with fencing and self-latching gates; and 5) fires/burns by use of smoke detectors and antiscald devices in shower heads and faucets.

Child abuse is a major contributor to childhood injuries from interpersonal violence—in 1986, an estimated 1.6 million children were abused or neglected. The occurrence of child abuse may be reduced through visits by public health nurses to mothers at high risk for child abuse. Other interventions include instructing parents at high risk for abuse in appropriate parenting skills; teaching children skills in identifying and reporting abusive situations; and conducting support groups for parents identified as being at high risk for child abuse.

An abridged version of *Childhood Injuries in the United States: A Report to Congress* was published in the June 1990 issue of *The American Journal of Diseases of Children* (4) and is available from the Division of Injury Control, Center for Environmental Health and Injury Control, CDC, Mailstop F36, Atlanta, Georgia 30333.

References
1. Committee on Trauma Research, Commission on Life Sciences, National Research Council, Institute of Medicine. Injury in America: a continuing public health problem. Washington, DC: National Academy Press, 1985.
2. Secretary of Health and Human Services. Childhood injuries in the United States: a report to Congress. Atlanta: US Department of Health and Human Services, Public Health Service, CDC, 1989.
3. Agran P, Castillo D, Winn D. Childhood motor vehicle occupant injuries. Am J Dis Child 1990;144:653–62.
4. CDC. Childhood injuries in the United States. Am J Dis Child 1990;144:627–46.
5. Azzara CV, Gallagher SS, Guyer B. The relative health care and social costs for specific causes of injury [Abstract]. In: Program and abstracts of the 113th annual meeting of the American Public Health Association. Washington, DC: American Public Health Association, 1985.
6. Rice DP, MacKenzie EJ, Jones AS, et al. The cost of injury in the United States: a report to Congress. San Francisco: Institute for Health and Aging, University of California; Injury Prevention Center, Johns Hopkins University, 1989.
7. Department of Health and Human Services, Department of Justice. Surgeon General's Workshop on Violence and Public Health: report. Washington, DC: US Department of Health and Human Services, Public Health Service, 1986; DHHS publication no. HRS-D-MC 86-1.
8. Alcohol, Drug Abuse, and Mental Health Administration. Report of the Secretary's Task Force on Youth Suicide. Rockville, Maryland: US Department of Health and Human Services, Public Health Service, 1989:115–28; DHHS publication no. (ADM)89-1624.

Deaths Due to Injury in the Home Among Persons Under 15 Years of Age, 1970–1984

Home mishaps caused one-fourth of all fatal injuries to children <15 years of age in the United States, with infants of both sexes and boys of all ages having the highest rates. Suffocation was the leading cause of fatal injuries among infants, whereas fires and burns were the main cause among children 1–14 years of age. The design of safer products and the use of functioning smoke detectors are among the most effective ways to prevent these types of deaths.

—MMWR Vol. 37/No. SS-1, February 1988, pp. 13–20

Deaths Due to Injury in the Home
Among Persons Under 15 Years of Age, 1970–1984

Daniel A. Pollock, M.D.
Daniel L. McGee, Ph.D.
Juan G. Rodriguez, M.D., M.P.H.
Division of Injury Epidemiology and Control
Center for Environmental Health and Injury Control

Introduction

Since 1950, mortality among children <15 years of age has declined substantially. Nearly all of this decline has been due to a reduction in the rate of deaths from natural causes (*1*). Injury has emerged as the leading cause of death among children 1-14 years of age, and incidents occurring in and around the home account for many of the fatal unintentional injuries to children (*2*).

The 1990 Objectives for the Nation include an objective to reduce the home injury fatality rate to no more than 5.0 per 100,000 for children <15 years of age. In 1978, the rate was 6.1 per 100,000 children <15 (*3*). This report is a review of the progress that has been made in meeting this 1990 objective, and it includes strategies to prevent children's deaths due to injury in the home.

Materials and Methods

Deaths. Data on the number of deaths occurring in the home were obtained from National Center for Health Statistics (NCHS) mortality tapes for the years 1970-1984. NCHS compiles mortality data from information recorded on death certificates. This information includes the decedent's age, race, sex, and date of death, and the underlying and contributory causes of death. The certificate also contains information on fatal injuries regarding the place of occurrence—for example, home, farm, street, or factory.

NCHS assigns the underlying cause of death and the place of occurrence of fatal injury according to the International Classification of Diseases (ICD) (*4*). The under-lying cause is selected from the ICD external causes of injury and poisoning (E codes), a classification system based on the circumstances and intentionality of the injury event. NCHS assigns a separate code for the place where the injury occurred. The definition for home as the place of occurrence includes apartment, boarding house, home premises, driveway to home, garage, yard, and swimming pool in private house or garden. This report provides data on deaths resulting from injury for which NCHS has coded the place of occurrence as "home."

NCHS has assigned a place-of-occurrence code for fatal unintentional injuries under both the ICD Eighth Revision (ICD-8) (in use 1968-1978) and the ICD Ninth Revision (ICD-9) (in use since the beginning of 1979). No place of occurrence is assigned to deaths due to suicide, homicide, and injuries of undetermined intention-ality. In this report, which describes trends for the period 1970-1984, the deaths discussed include only those due to injuries that were assigned a place-of-occurrence code according to ICD-9. (Place-of-occurrence codes are not assigned to unintentional injuries resulting from transport, medical and surgical procedures, or adverse reactions to drugs and medicinal substances in therapeutic use.)

Although death certifiers are instructed to enter on the death certificate the place where the injury occurred, the information they provide frequently does not allow vital statisticians to assign a specific code. The proportion of injury-related deaths with unspecified place-of-occurrence codes varies from year to year, and it was particularly high in 1981 and 1982—42.5% and 43.0%, respectively (NCHS unpublished data). In those 2 years, NCHS did not report place-of-occurrence data in its annual bound volumes of vital statistics (5,6). In this report, except for Table 4, data on home injury-related fatalities for 1981 and 1982 are excluded.

Population Data. Only residents <15 years of age are considered in this report. Population data used to calculate rates were taken from reports prepared by the Bureau of the Census (7-9).

Results

From 1970 through 1984 (excluding 1981 and 1982), an average of 3,212 persons <15 years of age died each year from injuries that occurred in the home. During this period, the number of deaths in this category decreased 38%, from 4,046 in 1970 to 2,527 in 1984 (Table 1). The home injury-related fatality rate among children <15 years of age decreased from 7.0 in 1970 to 5.0 (the 1990 objective target value) in 1983, and to 4.9 in 1984 (Figure 1).

TABLE 1. Deaths due to injury in the home among persons under 15 years of age, by year, United States, 1978-1984

Year	Total injury deaths*	Home injury deaths[†]	
		Number	**%Total**
1970	16,154	4,046	25.0
1971	16,077	3,791	23.6
1972	15,706	3,742	23.8
1973	15,629	3,467	22.2
1974	13,842	3,439	24.8
1975	13,186	3,196	24.2
1976	12,433	3,014	24.2
1977	12,279	2,971	24.2
1978	12,267	3,097	25.2
1979	11,428	2,929	25.6
1980	11,039	2,927	26.5
1983	9,597	2,605	27.1
1984	9,280	2,527	27.2

*Deaths for which the underlying cause assigned by NCHS was an injury or poisoning. The range of injury and poisoning codes (E800-E999) is the same in the eighth (ICD-8) and ninth (ICD-9) revisions of the International Classification of Diseases.

[†]Injury and poisoning deaths that are assigned a home place-of-occurrence code by ICD-9. In ICD-9, this code is used with categories E850-E869 and E880-E928. The corresponding ICD-8 categories are E850-E877 and E880-E929.

Source: National Center for Health Statistics (NCHS) mortality data tapes, 1970-1984.

FIGURE 1. Fatality rates due to injury in the home among persons under 15 years of age, by year, United States, 1970-1984

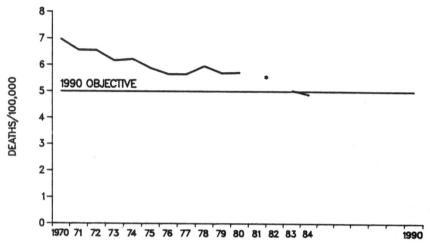

*Rates for 1981 and 1982 are omitted because the proportion of injury deaths with unspecified place-of-occurrence codes was particularly high in those years.

Table 2 presents fatality rates due to injury in the home by age group and sex for the years 1978 through 1984. The highest rate was for those <1 year of age. The rate for this age group declined from 16.8/100,000 in 1978 to 11.9/100,000 in 1984. This was the largest decrease in rate for any of the age groups. Males had a higher rate than females in all age groups.

Table 3 presents data on cause-specific categories. Fire and burn injuries (mainly from residential fires) were the largest category of home fatality, followed by drowning. After 1978, there was a decline in rate for every category, and the largest decreases occurred in the rates of falls and suffocation.

The pattern of cause-specific fatal injury in the home differed according to age group (Figure 2). In 1984, for children <1 year of age, suffocation was the leading cause of death, and no unintentional firearm fatalities were reported. For children 10-14 years of age, fire and burn injuries were the main cause of death, and firearms accounted for more than 30% of fatalities resulting from injuries that occurred in the home.

Table 4 shows the distribution of place-of-occurrence codes for fatal injuries to two age groups of children in the years 1978-1984. Children <5 years of age had a higher percentage of unspecified place-of-occurrence codes for each calendar year than did children 5-14 years of age. For both age groups, the data for 1981 and 1982 showed that the percentage of injuries with an unspecified place-of-occurrence code was one and a half to two times higher than the 1978-1980 levels.

TABLE 2. Deaths due to injury in the home among persons under 15 years of age, by age group, sex, and year, United States, 1978-1984

Age (years)		Deaths					
		Males		Females		Total	
		Number	Rate*	Number	Rate	Number	Rate
1978	<1	317	18.6	241	14.8	558	16.8
	1-4	845	13.3	566	9.3	1,411	11.4
	5-9	384	4.3	227	2.7	611	3.5
	10-14	362	3.7	155	1.7	517	2.7
	Total	1,908	7.2	1,189	4.7	3,097	6.0
1979	<1	278	15.9	225	13.4	503	14.7
	1-4	843	13.0	555	9.0	1,398	11.1
	5-9	349	4.0	211	2.5	560	3.3
	10-14	326	3.5	142	1.6	468	2.5
	Total	1,796	6.8	1,133	4.5	2,929	5.7
1980	<1	313	17.2	240	13.8	553	15.6
	1-4	838	12.7	563	8.9	1,401	10.9
	5-9	322	3.8	222	2.7	544	3.3
	10-14	292	3.1	137	1.5	429	2.4
	Total	1,765	6.7	1,162	4.6	2,927	5.7
1983	<1	262	13.9	196	10.9	458	12.4
	1-4	784	11.0	531	7.8	1,315	9.4
	5-9	250	3.0	193	2.4	443	2.7
	10-14	267	2.9	122	1.4	389	2.2
	Total	1,563	5.9	1,042	4.1	2,605	5.0
1984	<1	242	13.1	188	10.6	430	11.9
	1-4	768	10.6	474	6.8	1,242	8.7
	5-9	319	3.8	162	2.0	481	2.9
	10-14	270	3.0	104	1.2	374	2.1
	Total	1,599	6.0	928	3.7	2,527	4.9

*Deaths/100,000 children <15 years of age.

Source: National Center for Health Statistics mortality data tapes and Bureau of the Census population estimates.

Discussion

Mishaps occurring in and around the home cause one in four of the fatal injuries to children <15 years of age in the United States. From 1970 through 1984 (excluding 1981 and 1982), this proportion remained relatively constant, despite the decrease in the home injury fatality rates. Thus, although the 1990 objective of no more than 5.0 home injury deaths/100,000 children was met in 1983 and surpassed in 1984, a substantial proportion of children's injury mortality continues to result from injuries sustained in the home.

TABLE 3. Deaths due to injury in the home among persons under 15 years of age, by cause* and year, United States, 1978-1984

Year	Poisoning		Fall		Fire/Burn		Drowning		Suffocation		Firearm		Other	
	No.	Rate[†]	No.	Rate	No.	Rate	No.	Rate	No.	Rate	No.	Rate	No.	Rate
1978	119	0.23	179	0.34	1,524	2.93	426	0.82	489	0.94	201	0.39	159	0.31
1979	100	0.19	164	0.32	1,409	2.74	444	0.86	428	0.83	224	0.44	160	0.31
1980	93	0.18	146	0.28	1,378	2.69	463	0.90	472	0.92	211	0.41	164	0.32
1983	72	0.14	142	0.27	1,205	2.33	453	0.88	404	0.78	175	0.34	154	0.30
1984	79	0.15	87	0.17	1,243	2.40	382	0.74	400	0.77	181	0.35	155	0.30

*Cause-specific categories correspond to the following codes:

	ICD-8 (in use in 1978)	ICD-9 (in use since 1979)
Poisoning	E850-E877	E850-E869
Fall	E880-E887	E880-E888
Fire/Burn	E890-E899, E907, E923-E926	E890-E899, E907, E923-E926
Drowning	E910	E910
Suffocation	E911-E913	E911-E913
Firearm	E922	E922
Other	E900-E906, E908-E909, E914-E915, E916-E921, E927-E929	E900-E906, E908-E909, E914-E915, E916-E921, E927-E928

[†]Deaths/100,000 children <15 years of age.

Source: National Center for Health Statistics mortality data tapes and Bureau of the Census population estimates.

In this study, fatality rates varied by age and sex, with infants of both sexes and males of all age groups having the highest rates. Suffocation was the leading cause of home injury-related fatalities among children <1 year of age, and fires and burns were the main cause of these fatalities among children from 1 through 14 years of age.

Many injury control strategies have been implemented or made available to prevent childhood deaths from injuries in the home (2,10,11). The reduction of childhood suffocations has been attributed to the regulations and standards pertaining to the design of consumer products (12,13). The U.S. Fire Administration estimates that the use of smoke detectors decreases by half the risk of dying in a house fire (14). Although the percentage of U.S. homes with smoke detectors has increased steadily since the early 1970s, one community inspection showed that nearly 30% of the installed detectors were nonfunctioning (15). Proper installation and frequent testing are necessary to ensure adequate protection (16). Other measures to prevent fatal home fires include automatic fire-suppressant sprinkler systems and self-extinguishing cigarettes (17,18).

TABLE 4. Deaths due to injury in the home among persons under 15 years of age, by age group, place of occurrence, and year, United States, 1978-1984

| Year | Deaths | Under 5 years | | | 5-14 years | | |
| | | Place of occurrence | | | Place of occurrence | | |
		Home	Other	Unspecified	Home	Other	Unspecified
1978	No.	1,969	467	649	1,128	1,196	393
	%	63.8	15.1	21.0	41.5	44.0	14.5
1979	No.	1,901	470	499	1,028	1,110	301
	%	66.2	16.4	17.4	42.1	45.5	12.3
1980	No.	1,954	529	456	973	1,039	209
	%	66.5	18.0	15.5	43.8	46.8	9.4
1981	No.	1,595	344	844	828	639	597
	%	57.3	12.4	30.3	40.1	31.0	28.9
1982	No.	1,503	342	835	797	633	544
	%	56.1	12.8	31.2	40.4	32.1	27.6
1983	No.	1,773	490	394	832	856	199
	%	66.7	18.4	14.8	44.1	45.4	10.5
1984	No.	1,672	375	345	855	714	181
	%	69.9	15.7	14.4	48.9	40.8	10.3

*Source: National Center for Health Statistics mortality data tapes.

FIGURE 2. Distribution of fatalities due to injury in the home among persons under 15 years of age, by cause and age group (years), United States, 1984

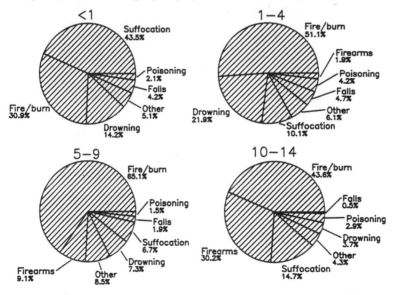

Much of the decline in childhood poisoning fatalities in the home has been ascribed to interventions aimed at reducing the incidence of potentially lethal ingestions (*19*). An industry-government conference in 1966 led to the restriction of children's aspirin to 36 tablets per container, and the Poison Prevention Packaging Act of 1970 resulted in safety packaging of aspirin and other products (*20,21*). Steps to promote further risk reduction include technical improvements in child-resistant containers and instruction in the proper use of child-resistant packaging for persons who have frequent contact with children (*22*).

The rate of child drownings in fresh water is lower in communities that require swimming pool fencing than it is in communities without such regulations (*23*). Swimming lessons for infants are popular; still, controlled studies are needed to clarify benefits and risks (*24*).

Some prevention efforts directed at specific types of falls in childhood have proved effective (*25*). Identifying home hazards and providing free, easily installed window guards led to a reduction of deaths due to falls among children living in apartment buildings in New York City (*26*).

Unintentional firearm-related deaths among children can be reduced by interventions such as improving the design of safety catches so that firearms will not be discharged inadvertently (*27*).

Although the rate of children's fatalities due to injury in the home has declined in recent years, surveillance continues to be important in view of the magnitude of the problem and the need to evaluate the efficacy of intervention strategies. The use of NCHS mortality data for these purposes is limited by three constraints. First, the data tapes are not available for public use until at least 18 months after the end of the data year (*28*). Second, specific place-of-occurrence codes for all deaths resulting from injury are not available. This limitation impedes the determination of incidence and trends for particular calendar years and age groups. For example, although incidents occurring in the home are the leading cause of injury deaths among children <5 years old, a relatively high percentage of place-of-occurrence codes are unspecified for this age group (Table 4) (*2*). Third, NCHS mortality data provide important demographic information, but they do not contain details about the circumstances of the injury beyond the external cause and the place of occurrence. Injury events usually involve a complex interaction of many elements that are not fully described by means of the current external-cause coding system (*29*).

References
1. National Center for Health Statistics. Health: United States, 1982. Washington, DC: US Department of Health and Human Services, 1982.
2. Dershewitz RA, Christopherson ER. Childhood household safety: an overview. Am J Dis Child 1984;138:85-8.
3. US Department of Health and Human Services, Public Health Service. Promoting health/ preventing disease: objectives for the nation. Washington, DC: US Department of Health and Human Services, 1980.
4. World Health Organization. Manual of the international statistical classification of diseases, injuries, and causes of death, ninth revision. Geneva: World Health Organization, 1977.
5. National Center for Health Statistics. Vital statistics of the United States, 1981: II. Mortality, part A. Washington, DC: US Department of Health and Human Services, 1986.
6. National Center for Health Statistics. Vital Statistics of the United States, 1982: II. Mortality, part A. Washington, DC: US Department of Health and Human Services, 1986.

7. US Department of Commerce, Bureau of the Census. Current population reports: preliminary estimates of the population of the United States, by age, sex, and race: 1970 to 1981. Washington, DC: US Department of Commerce, 1982. (Series P-25, no. 917).

8. US Department of Commerce, Bureau of the Census. Current population reports: estimates of the population of the United States, by age, sex, and race: 1980 to 1983. Washington, DC: US Department of Commerce, 1984. (Series P-25, no. 949).

9. US Department of Commerce, Bureau of the Census. Current population reports: estimates of the population of the United States, by age, sex, and race: 1980 to 1986. Washington, DC: US Department of Commerce, 1987. (Series P-25, no. 1000).

10. Gallagher SS, Hunter P, Guyer B. A home injury prevention program for children. Pediatr Clin North Am 1985;32:95-112.

11. Rivara FP. Traumatic deaths of children in the United States: currently available prevention strategies. Pediatrics 1985;75:456-62.

12. Baker SP, Fisher RS. Childhood asphyxiation by choking or suffocation. JAMA 1980;244:1343-6.

13. Kraus JF. Effectiveness of measures to prevent unintentional deaths of infants and children from suffocation and strangulation. Public Health Rep 1985;100:231-40.

14. Hall JR. A decade of detectors: measuring the effect. Fire J 1985;79:37-43,78.

15. CDC. Prevalence of smoke detectors in private residences—Dekalb County, Georgia, 1985. MMWR 1986;35:445-8.

16. US Consumer Product Safety Commission. What you should know about smoke detectors. Washington DC: US Consumer Product Safety Commission, 1983.

17. US Fire Administration. An ounce of prevention. Washington, DC: Federal Emergency Management Agency, 1983.

18. McGuire A. Cigarettes and fire deaths. NY State J Med 1983;83:1296-8.

19. Rodriguez JG, Sattin RW. Epidemiology of childhood poisonings leading to hospitalization in the United States, 1979-1983. Am J Prev Med 1987;3:164-70.

20. Clarke A, Walton WW. Effect of safety packaging on aspirin ingestion by children. Pediatrics 1979;63:687-93.

21. Walton WW. An evaluation of the Poison Prevention Packaging Act. Pediatrics 1982;69:363-70.

22. CDC. Unintentional ingestions of prescription drugs in children under five years old. MMWR 1987;36:124-6,131-2.

23. Pearn JH, Wong RYK, Brown J, et al. Drowning and near drowning involving children: a five-year total population study from the city and county of Honolulu. Am J Public Health 1979;69:450-4.

24. Pearn JH. Current controversies in child accident prevention: an analysis of some areas of dispute in the prevention of child trauma. Aust NZ J Med 1985;15:782-7.

25. Garretson LK, Gallagher SS. Falls in children and youth. Pediatr Clin North Am 1985;32:153-62.

26. Spiegel CN, Lindaman FC. Children can't fly: a program to prevent childhood morbidity and mortality from window falls. Am J Public Health 1977;67:1143-7.

27. Wintemute GJ, Teret SP, Kraus JF, et al. When children shoot children: 88 unintended deaths in California. JAMA 1987;257:3107-9.

28. Pearce ND. National Center for Health Statistics. Data systems of the National Center for Health Statistics. Hyattsville, Maryland: US Department of Health and Human Services, 1981. (Vital and health statistics; series 1; no. 16).

29. Langley J. The International Classification of Diseases codes for describing injuries and the circumstances surrounding injuries: a critical comment and suggestions for improvement. Accid Anal Prev 1982;14:195-7.

Unintentional Firearm-Related Fatalities Among Children and Teenagers — United States, 1982–1988

Interventions to reduce morbidity and death from unintentional firearm-related injuries among children and teenagers must emphasize locked and separate storage of weapons and ammunition in the home.

—MMWR Vol. 41/No. 25, June 26, 1992, pp. 442–5, 451

Unintentional Firearm-Related Fatalities
Among Children and Teenagers — United States, 1982-1988

In 1988, gunshot wounds were the eighth leading cause of unintentional injury deaths among persons in all age groups in the United States and the third leading cause of such deaths among children and teenagers aged 10–19 years (1). From 1982 through 1988, 3607 children and teenagers aged 0–19 years died from unintentional firearm-related injuries, constituting 32% of all unintentional firearm-related deaths. Of those, 81% occurred among 10–19-year-olds. This article describes a case report of an unintentional firearm-related death of a teenager and summarizes an analysis of demographic and regional differences in unintentional firearm-related mortality among children and teenagers from 1982 through 1988.

Case Report

In a large metropolitan area in the southern United States, two brothers were playing in their home with two friends while the boys' parents were at work. Initially, they played in the boys' bedroom using the bunk beds and bedspreads to build "forts"; they also engaged in gun play using plastic toy guns. Later, they divided into two teams to play hide-and-seek. One of the boys, a 13-year-old, hid in his parents' bedroom where he found his father's 12-gauge shotgun stored under the bed. The shotgun was kept in the house for protection; the boy did not know it was loaded. When his friend, also aged 13 years, entered the room looking for him, the boy who was hiding inadvertently discharged the gun, killing his friend.

Analysis of National Mortality Data

Demographic and regional differences in firearm-related mortality were examined using mortality data compiled by CDC's National Center for Health Statistics. Unintentional firearm-related deaths were identified by the *International Classification of Diseases, Ninth Revision*, code E922. Classification of counties as metropolitan and nonmetropolitan is based on metropolitan statistical areas designated by the U.S. Office of Management and Budget in 1982.

For males aged 10–19 years, the unintentional firearm-related death rate was 10 times that for females (2.0 per 100,000 versus 0.2 per 100,000 children). Males aged 15–19 years were at higher risk (2.4 per 100,000) than were males in any other age group. The risk for dying from an unintentional gunshot wound was similar for black and white children and teenagers aged 10–19 years.

Children and teenagers living in the South* were at greatest risk for dying from an unintentional gunshot wound; those living in the Northeast[†] were at lowest risk (Table 1). Within regions, white males aged 15–19 years were at greatest risk in the South; in all other regions, death rates were highest for black male teenagers. Overall, children and teenagers living in nonmetropolitan regions were more than twice as likely to die from an unintentional gunshot wound as those living in metropolitan areas; however, the rate ratio in nonmetropolitan and metropolitan areas was 1.4 for black males aged 10–14 years and 1.1 for black males aged 15–19 years (Table 2).

Reported by: Unintentional Injuries Section, Epidemiology Br, and Biometrics Br, Div of Injury Control, National Center for Environmental Health and Injury Control, CDC.

---

*South Atlantic, East South Central, and West South Central regions.
[†]New England and Middle Atlantic regions.

TABLE 1. Number and rate* of unintentional firearm-related deaths, by region, age, race, and sex — United States, 1982–1988

Age group (yrs)	Northeast[†] No.	Rate	South[§] No.	Rate	Midwest[¶] No.	Rate	West** No.	Rate	Total No.	Rate
10–14										
White										
Male	71	0.7	470	2.9	183	1.4	167	1.7	891	1.8
Female	11	0.1	52	0.3	25	0.2	26	0.3	114	0.2
Black										
Male	1	0.1	65	1.3	19	1.0	14	1.9	99	1.1
Female	1	0.1	17	0.3	4	0.2	3	0.4	25	0.3
Total[††]	84	0.4	606	1.4	236	0.8	222	1.0	1148	1.0
15–19										
White										
Male	132	1.1	630	3.6	271	1.8	273	2.5	1306	2.4
Female	14	0.1	57	0.3	19	0.1	20	0.2	110	0.2
Black										
Male	28	1.5	125	2.4	52	2.7	54	6.3	259	2.6
Female	2	0.1	18	0.3	3	0.2	8	1.0	31	0.3
Total[††]	177	0.6	840	1.8	354	1.1	391	1.5	1762	1.3

*Per 100,000 children and teenagers.
[†]New England and Middle Atlantic regions.
[§]South Atlantic, East South Central, and West South Central regions.
[¶]East North Central and West North Central regions.
**Mountain and Pacific regions.
[††]Includes all races.

TABLE 2. Number and rate* of unintentional firearm-related deaths, by metropolitan area, age, race, and sex — United States, 1982–1988

Age group (yrs)	Metropolitan area No.	Rate	Nonmetropolitan area No.	Rate
10–14				
White				
Male	473	1.3	418	3.1
Female	63	0.2	51	0.4
Black				
Male	74	1.0	25	1.4
Female	16	0.2	9	0.5
Total[†]	630	0.7	518	1.7
15–19				
White				
Male	773	1.9	533	3.8
Female	59	0.2	51	0.4
Black				
Male	204	2.6	55	2.8
Female	26	0.3	5	0.3
Total[†]	1081	1.1	681	2.1

*Per 100,000 children and teenagers.
[†]Includes all races.

Editorial Note: Despite recent declines in unintentional firearm-related mortality (*1,2*), such injuries continue to disproportionately affect youth nationwide. Unintentional firearm-related injuries are also a major cause of morbidity. For example, a recent report by the General Accounting Office (GAO) estimated that, in 10 U.S. cities during 1989 and 1990, the ratio of nonfatal to fatal unintentional gunshot wounds was 105 to 1 for all age groups combined (*3*). Although the findings of the GAO report cannot be generalized to the entire United States, they underscore the public health impact of unintentional firearm-related injuries.

The high rates of unintentional firearm-related mortality for children and teenagers living in southern and western regions of the country are consistent with the findings of previous reports (*1*). Although most reports have demonstrated a higher death rate for those living in rural areas (*1,4*), one study in Cleveland, Ohio, found rates were higher in urban areas than in the suburbs (*5*).

The findings in this report indicate that, although death rates of unintentional firearm-related injuries were generally higher for children and teenagers living in nonmetropolitan areas, death rates for black males in metropolitan areas approached those in nonmetropolitan areas. Risk factors, such as access to firearms and per capita income, may have a differential impact on unintentional firearm-related mortality. For example, the availability of firearms has been directly associated with unintentional gunshot wounds (*5*), and the relation between per capita income of the area of residence and unintentional firearm-related mortality varies inversely (*1*).

Reduction of morbidity and mortality from unintentional firearm-related injuries among children and teenagers must emphasize limiting access to loaded weapons. Specific behavioral characteristics associated with adolescence, such as impulsivity, feelings of invincibility, and curiosity about firearms, place adolescents at particularly high risk for firearm-related injuries (*6*).

One of the national health objectives for the year 2000 is to reduce by 20% the proportion of households with inappropriately stored weapons (objective 7.11) (*7*). This objective is consistent with the findings of several studies indicating that most unintentional firearm-related deaths involving children occur at a residence (*4,8,9*) and involve inappropriately stored weapons (*9*). Appropriate storage should include locked and separate storage of weapons and ammunition. In Florida and California, legislation has been enacted to make adults legally responsible for inappropriate storage.

Modifying firearms and ammunition to render them less lethal has also been advocated as a prevention strategy (*1,10*). The addition of child-proof safety devices would prevent children aged <6 years from discharging a firearm, and the use of loading indicators could prevent an estimated 23% of all unintentional firearm-related deaths (*3*). Regulation to control the amount of gunpowder and the shape and jacketing of ammunition may reduce the severity of nonfatal firearm-related injuries (*1,10*).

References
1. Baker SP, O'Neill B, Ginsburg MJ, Li G. The injury fact book. 2nd ed. New York: Oxford University Press, 1992.
2. Wood NP Jr, Mercy JA. Unintentional firearm-related fatalities, 1970–1984. In: CDC surveillance summaries, February 1988. MMWR 1988;37(no. SS-1):47–52.
3. US General Accounting Office. Accidental shootings: many deaths and injuries caused by firearms could be prevented—report to the Chairman, Subcommittee on Antitrust, Monopolies, and Business Rights, Committee on the Judiciary, House of Representatives. Washington, DC: US General Accounting Office, 1991; report no. GAO/PEMD-91-9.

4. Keck NJ, Istre GR, Coury DL, Jordan F, Eaton AP. Characteristics of fatal gunshot wounds in the home in Oklahoma: 1982–1983. Am J Dis Child 1988;142:623–6.
5. Rushforth NB, Hirsch CS, Ford AB, Adelson L. Accidental firearm fatalities in a metropolitan county (1958–1973). Am J Epidemiol 1975;100:499–505.
6. Committee on Adolescence, American Academy of Pediatrics. Firearms and adolescents. AAP News 1992;(January):20–1.
7. Public Health Service. Healthy people 2000: national health promotion and disease prevention objectives—full report, with commentary. Washington, DC: US Department of Health and Human Services, Public Health Service, 1991; DHHS publication no. (PHS)91-50212.
8. Wintemute GJ, Kraus JF, Teret SP, Wright MA. Unintentional firearm deaths in California. J Trauma 1989;29:457–61.
9. Beaver BL, Moore VL, Peclet M, Haller JA Jr, Smialek J, Hill JL. Characteristics of pediatric firearm fatalities. J Pediatr Surg 1990;25:97–100.
10. Christoffel KK. Toward reducing pediatric injuries from firearms: charting a legislative and regulatory course. Pediatrics 1991;88:294–305.

Premature Mortality Due to Unintentional Injuries — United States, 1984

In 1984, motor vehicle traffic crashes were the leading cause of both deaths and years of potential life lost resulting from unintentional injuries. Reductions of fatalities among motor vehicle occupants and pedestrians depend on a variety of interventions designed to alter the human and environmental factors affecting motor vehicle crashes. Also in 1984, poisonings, drownings, falls, and fires combined were responsible for 13,481 deaths and 498,858 years of potential life lost.

—MMWR Vol. 36/No. 49, December 18, 1987, pp. 814–5

Premature Mortality Due to Unintentional Injuries — United States, 1984

Unintentional injuries are the leading cause of years of potential life lost (YPLL) before the age of 65. In 1985, unintentional injuries (E800-949)* accounted for over 2.2 million YPLL, or 19% of all YPLL. Unintentional injuries were also the leading cause of YPLL in 1983 and 1984 (1).

For this analysis, National Center for Health Statistics (NCHS) mortality data for 1984, the latest year for which detailed data are available, were used to determine the number of deaths associated with unintentional injury and the related YPLL. Population data, based on the 1984 U.S. Bureau of the Census estimates, were used to calculate age- and cause-specific YPLL rates.

In 1984, motor vehicle traffic crashes (E810-819), which caused 39,228 deaths, were the leading cause of both YPLL and deaths resulting from unintentional injuries. Injuries to passenger vehicle occupants are the major cause of deaths due to motor vehicle crashes and cause one out of every three deaths from all causes among 15-to 19-year-old males (2). Deaths from drowning (E910), fire and flames (E890-899), poisoning (E850-869), falls (E880-888), unintentional discharge of firearms (E922), and choking on food or objects (E911-912) were also leading causes of YPLL in 1984.

Fatalities caused by nontraffic motor vehicle crashes involving off-the-road vehicles, such as snowmobiles and all-terrain vehicles, and fatalities due to air and water transportation remained among the ten unintentional injuries that cause the largest number of deaths and YPLL (Table 1). For all unintentional injuries, the rate of YPLL for males was between 1.7 and 8.9 times greater (depending on the unintentional injury) than that for females. This difference was greatest for fatal injuries involving air transportion.

TABLE 1. Deaths and years of potential life lost (YPLL) due to unintentional injuries before age 65 — United States, 1984

Cause of Mortality (ICD, 9th Revision)	Deaths	YPLL
Motor Vehicle, Traffic (E810-819)	39,228	1,387,534
Poisonings (E850-869)	4,244	130,632
Drowning (E910)	3,982	162,656
Falls (E880-888)	3,168	72,889
Fire and Flames (E890-899)	2,087	132,681
Firearms (E922)	1,538	58,579
Choking (E911-912)	1,354	38,342
Air Transport (E840-845)	1,187	32,151
Water Transport (E830-838)	1,027	32,641
Motor Vehicle, Nontraffic (E820-825)	901	35,978

In 1984, fatalities involving pedestrians were the second leading cause of motor vehicle traffic deaths and constituted about 14% of all fatalities associated with motor vehicle traffic incidents. A total of 5,652 persons were killed in pedestrian incidents, and a resultant 195,586 years of potential life were lost. White males had a YPLL rate of 120.7/100,000 population for pedestrian fatalities, and black males had a rate of

---

*Based on the International Classification of Diseases, 9th Revision, Supplementary Classification of External Causes of Injury and Poisoning.

225.3/100,000. The rates for white and black females showed a similar difference. Although the age-specific fatality rate for pedestrians was high for children under age 5, it was highest for adults 15-29 years of age and for those over 50. Children under 10 contributed 26% of the YPLL due to pedestrian fatalities.

Reported by: Program Development and Implementation Br, Div of Injury Epidemiology and Control, Center for Environmental Health and Injury Control, CDC.

Editorial Note: Alcohol is the single most frequently found human factor in fatal crashes *(3,4)*. A 1982 study of 46 motor vehicle crashes in Fulton County, Georgia, in which the drivers' blood alcohol concentrations (BACs) were measured showed that, in 39 (85%) of the crashes, at least one of the drivers involved was legally intoxicated. Drivers who had been drinking were involved in 42 (91%) of the crashes. Thirty-two (82%) of the legally intoxicated drivers were at least 25 years old, and 30 (77%) were male *(5)*.

Deaths involving pedestrians represent the second largest category of motor vehicle deaths. Males account for 70% of pedestrian fatalities in all age groups. Two-thirds of all pedestrian deaths occur in urban areas. Alcohol plays a major role in adult pedestrian fatalities *(3,4)*. Almost half of all fatally injured adult pedestrians have BACs $\geq$0.1%, and more than 50% of all fatally injured pedestrians in the 20- to 64-year age group have BACs $\geq$0.1%. For persons killed in motor vehicle crashes, the percentage of elevated BAC declines after age 40.

Reductions of motor vehicle occupant and pedestrian fatalities depend on a variety of interventions designed to alter the human and environmental factors affecting motor vehicle crashes. Interventions that could reduce human factors in motor vehicle crashes include public awareness and legal enforcement actions designed to deter alcohol use by drivers and pedestrians and special educational efforts directed toward these two groups. Studies of the cost-effectiveness of possible engineering changes, such as altering vehicle and highway design and constructing barriers to physically separate pedestrians and vehicles, may reveal some other important interventions.

References
1. Centers for Disease Control. Premature mortality due to unintentional injuries—United States, 1983. MMWR 1986;35:353-6.
2. Baker SP, O'Neill B, Karpf RS. The injury fact book. Lexington, Massachusetts: Lexington Books, 1984.
3. Waller JA. Injury control: a guide to the causes and prevention of trauma. Lexington, Massachusetts: Lexington Books, 1985:211.
4. Haddon W Jr, Valien P, McCarroll JR, Umberger CJ. A controlled investigation of the characteristics of adult pedestrians fatally injured by motor vehicles in Manhattan. J Chronic Dis 1961;14:655-78.
5. Centers for Disease Control. Alcohol and fatal injuries—Fulton County, Georgia, 1982. MMWR 1983;32:573-6.

Premature Mortality Due to Unintentional Injuries — United States, 1983

Injury exacts an enormous toll in the United States, causing more than 140,000 deaths and over 3.5 million years of potential life lost per year. The five leading causes of years of potential life lost are motor vehicle crashes, drownings, fire and flames, poisonings, and falls.

—MMWR Vol. 35/No. 22, June 6, 1986, pp. 353–6

Premature Mortality Due to Unintentional Injuries — United States, 1983

As life expectancy has increased in the United States, the leading causes of death have shifted to those diseases occurring late in life, such as heart disease, cancer, and stroke. Mortality rates have long been used to measure the magnitude of these diseases and to determine resource allocation in public health. However, this traditional measure of mortality does not provide the information needed to compare the amount of premature mortality by cause of death. In 1950, an index was proposed that expressed deaths in terms of years of life lost (YLL) to complement conventional death rates (1). However, the YLL index was little used during the 1950s and 1960s. A 1965 study noted that injuries caused a significant loss of years of life and that the allocation of health resources must consider not only the number of deaths by cause but also by age (2). During the 1970s and early 1980s, the YLL index became an accepted tool for state and local health planners (3). In 1982, CDC began reporting years of potential life lost before age 65 years (YPLL) in Table V of the *MMWR*. The YPLL index draws attention to potentially preventable mortality occurring early in life.

Table V. Estimated years of potential life lost before age 65 and cause-specific mortality, by cause of death — United States, 1984

Cause of mortality (Ninth Revision ICD)	Years of potential life lost by persons dying in 1984*	Cause-specific mortality[†] (rate/100,000)
ALL CAUSES (Total)	11,761,000	866.7
Unintentional injuries[§] (E800-E949)	2,308,000	40.1
Malignant neoplasms (140-208)	1,803,000	191.6
Diseases of the heart (390-398, 402, 404-429)	1,563,000	324.4
Suicide, homicide (E950-E978)	1,247,000	20.6
Congenital anomalies (740-759)	684,000	5.6
Prematurity[¶] (765, 769)	470,000	3.5
Sudden infant death syndrome (798)	314,000	2.4
Cerebrovascular diseases (430-438)	266,000	65.6
Chronic liver diseases and cirrhosis (571)	233,000	11.3
Pneumonia and influenza (480-487)	163,000	25.0
Chronic obstructive pulmonary diseases (490-496)	123,000	29.8
Diabetes mellitus (250)	119,000	15.6

*For details of calculation, see footnotes for Table V, *MMWR* 1986;35:27.
[†]Cause-specific mortality rates as reported in the MVSR are compiled from a 10% sample of all deaths.
[§]Equivalent to accidents and adverse effects.
[¶]Category derived from disorders relating to short gestation and respiratory distress syndrome.

Unintentional injuries are the leading cause of YPLL. In 1984, they accounted for 2,308,000 YPLL, or about 19.6% of all YPLL (see Table V, page 365). Overall, unintentional injuries (E800-E949)* accounted for 2,277,000 YPLL in 1983, or about 19.4% of all YPLL. This report focuses on the 10 leading causes of YPLL due to unintentional injury for 1983, the last year for which complete data are available.

For this report, age- and cause-specific mortality data obtained from the National Center for Health Statistics (NCHS) were used to determine the number of deaths and to calculate the YPLL for each cause of unintentional injury death in the United States during 1983. Population estimates from the U.S. Bureau of the Census were used to calculate YPLL rates.

Among unintentional injuries, motor vehicle traffic crashes (E810-E819) are the leading cause of both YPLL and deaths (Figure 1). Among all other causes of death, motor vehicle traffic crashes rank only below malignant neoplasms and diseases of the heart for YPLL. The remaining 10 leading causes of YPLL from unintentional injuries, in order, are: drownings (E910),[†] fire and flames (E890-E899), poisonings (E850-E869), falls (E880-E888), firearms (E922), choking on food or object (E911-E912), water transport (E830-E838), air transport (E840-E845), and motor vehicle nontraffic crashes (E820-E825).

The rank order of the cause-specific numbers of deaths is the same as that of YPLL, except for fire and flames (fourth instead of third) and water transport (ninth instead of eighth).

---

*Based on The International Classification of Diseases, 9th Revision, Supplementary Classification of External Cause of Injury.
[†]Includes those not related to water transport.

FIGURE 1. Years of potential life lost (YPLL) and number of deaths for the 10 leading causes of unintentional injury YPLL — United States, 1983

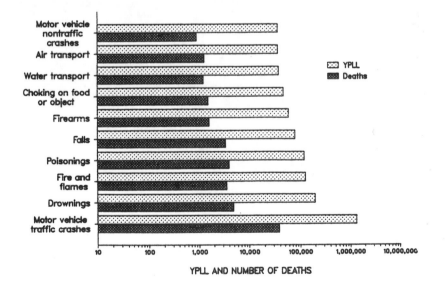

Crude YPLL rates per 100,000 population and average YPLL per death (equivalent to 65 minus the average age at death) vary by each of the 10 leading causes of unintentional injury YPLL and by the sex of the victim (Table 1). The variation by sex in the YPLL rates is measured in the YPLL rate ratios. Males have higher YPLL rates than females for each of the listed unintentional injury causes of death. The highest YPLL rate ratios for males compared with females are for deaths due to water transport and deaths due to firearms, whereas the lowest

TABLE 1. Years of potential life lost (YPLL) rates per 100,000 population, YPLL rate ratios, and average YPLL per death, by the 10 leading causes of unintentional injury YPLL and by sex — United States, 1983.

Cause of death	YPLL rate	(YPLL rate ratio[*])	Average YPLL per death
Motor vehicle traffic crashes			
Male	953.1		35.1
Female	334.3	(2.9)	34.6
Drownings[†]			
Male	156.7		39.9
Female	33.7	(4.7)	43.9
Fire and flames			
Male	73.9		33.7
Female	47.8	(1.5)	38.4
Poisonings			
Male	81.7		30.4
Female	33.4	(2.4)	29.1
Falls			
Male	59.5		23.6
Female	16.1	(3.7)	21.6
Firearms			
Male	49.0		36.8
Female	7.8	(6.3)	38.2
Choking on food or object			
Male	26.8		27.7
Female	14.5	(1.8)	29.5
Air transport			
Male	29.3		28.0
Female	5.9	(5.0)	31.5
Water transport			
Male	32.7		30.6
Female	3.8	(8.6)	34.5
Motor vehicle nontraffic crashes			
Male	26.6		39.1
Female	8.3	(3.2)	45.8

[*]For males compared with females within each cause-specific category.

[†]Includes those not related to water transport.

are for deaths due to fire and flames and deaths due to choking on food or object. Except for motor vehicle traffic crashes, poisonings. and falls, the average YPLL per death is higher for females than males. The highest average YPLL per death is for that associated with motor vehicle nontraffic crashes for females, and the lowest is for that associated with falls for females.

Both YPLL and mortality rates highlight the importance of injuries as a health problem among children. Annually, about 10,000 children aged 1-14 years die from injuries (4). Injuries account for more deaths among children than any disease. The six leading causes of unintentional injury death among children are: motor vehicles, drownings, fire and flames, choking on food or object, firearms, and falls (5). About 40% of motor vehicle deaths among children involved the child as a pedestrian (4). Considered as a separate cause of deaths among children, pedestrian death is the third leading cause of unintentional injury death after deaths among motor vehicle occupants and deaths due to drowning.

Reported by Div of Injury Epidemiology and Control, Center for Environmental Health, CDC.

Editorial Note: Injury exacts an enormous toll in the United States, causing more than 140,000 deaths and over 3.5 million years of potential life lost per year (see Table V, page 365). Intentional injuries result from interpersonal or self-inflicted violence and include homicide, assaults, suicide and suicide attempts, child abuse, and rape. Unintentional injuries include those resulting from motor vehicle collisions, falls, fires, poisonings, and drownings. Injuries occur during work and include unintentional trauma (e.g., motor vehicle-related injuries, falls, and electrocutions) and intentional injuries. One in every three Americans suffers an injury each year, and 80,000 persons suffer permanent disabling injuries from brain or spinal cord trauma (6). Direct and indirect costs of injury are estimated at $75-$100 billion per year.

The use of YPLL has become a mainstay in the evaluation of the impact of injuries on public health. Although YPLL is a valuable index in analyzing various causes of injury mortality, this report also includes YPLL rates, YPLL rate ratios, and average YPLL per death. The use of YPLL rates allows comparison of YLL between different populations. For each of the 10 leading causes of unintentional injury YPLL, males have a higher rate of YPLL than females. These higher rates in males may reflect a greater involvement in hazardous activities, in use of alcohol (4), and in risk-taking behavior. However, the use of average YPLL per death shows that, among those who die from unintentional injuries, females, on average, are dying at a younger age than males for each of the 10 leading causes of unintentional injury YPLL, except for motor vehicle traffic crashes, poisonings, and falls. Persons are dying from drownings, motor vehicle nontraffic crashes, and firearms at a younger age, on average, than from the other leading causes of unintentional injury YPLL.

When injuries are studied epidemiologically, many opportunities for prevention may become evident. What is known about host, agent, and environment can be translated into programmatically sound interventions that reduce injury morbidity and mortality. A project of the Carter Center of Emory University entitled, "Closing the Gap," examined the impact of the injury problem and its potential reduction by applying existing scientific and technical knowledge (7). The Carter Center estimates that, by applying broad-based mixed strategies, motor vehicle-related fatalities and injuries could be reduced by about 75% (8). About 23,000 deaths per year result from unintentional injuries that occur in the home (8). The Carter Center estimates that targeted interventions could reduce home injuries by about 50% (8). Appropriately targeted interventions also could reduce by about 25% all fatal and serious injuries in which alcohol is an important factor (8).

Past and current research and surveillance efforts have identified many prevention strategies to be applied and evaluated, and a growing number of state and local public health agencies and other organizations are now in the process of meeting this challenge. State agencies, in particular, can assume several responsibilities in injury prevention, including: (1) coordinating their activities with local agencies, academic institutions, and private entities; (2) conducting injury surveillance; (3) developing intervention plans with other involved groups; (4) providing information to the public; and (5) providing technical advice on legislative proposals needed to support injury-control efforts.

References
1. Haenszel W. A standardized rate for mortality defined in units of lost years of life. Am J Public Health 1950;40:17-26.
2. Stickle G. What priority, human life? Am J Public Health 1965;55:1692-8.
3. Perloff JD, LeBailly SA, Kletke PR, Budetti PP, Connelly JP. Premature death in the United States: years of life lost and health priorities. J Pub Health Policy 1984;5:167-184.
4. Baker SP, O'Neill B, Karpf RS. The injury fact book. Lexington, Massachusetts: Lexington Books, 1984:20.
5. National Safety Council. Accident facts, 1985. Chicago: National Safety Council, 1985.
6. Institute of Medicine and National Research Council. Injury in America. Washington, D.C.: National Academy Press, 1985.
7. Foege WH, Amler RW, White CC. Closing the gap. Report of the Carter Center health policy consultation. JAMA 1985;254:1355-8.
8. Smith GS. Measuring the gap for unintentional injuries: the Carter Center health policy project. Public Health Rep 1985;100:565-8.

Injuries in an Indian Community — Cherokee, North Carolina

Among American Indians and Alaskan Natives, the combined unintentional and intentional injury mortality rate is three times the rate for the general U.S. population. The Tribal Council, the Community Injury Control Committee, and other community leaders and organizations have planned interventions to decrease sports-related injuries, improve roads, reduce intentional injuries, and encourage the use of seat belts and child-restraint seats.

—MMWR Vol. 36/No. 47, December 4, 1987, pp. 779-81

Injuries in an Indian Community — Cherokee, North Carolina

The American Indian/Alaskan Native population experiences a disproportionate amount of morbidity and mortality from injuries (1). To address this public health problem, the Cherokee Service Unit of the Indian Health Service studied the injury morbidity and mortality of the Eastern Band of the Cherokee Indians in North Carolina. Investigators reviewed the emergency room (ER) records from the Cherokee Indian Hospital for the period July 1, 1984, through June 30, 1985.* This ER is the only emergency care facility within the 56,000 acres of the rural Cherokee Indian Reservation, located near the Smoky Mountain National Park.

During this period, 1,448 injured persons visited the ER, for an incidence rate of 240 visits per 1,000 population. Sixty-three percent of those who sought care were male. The male to female injury rate ratio was 1.6:1. Injury rates for males exceeded rates for females in all age groups up to age 40 (Figure 1). After age 40, females had a higher injury rate than males. Rates for males peaked at 10-19 years of age and declined sharply thereafter. For females, rates generally decreased with increasing age.

FIGURE 1. Age- and sex-specific injury rates, by age group — Cherokee Reservation, Cherokee, North Carolina, July 1, 1984–June 30, 1985

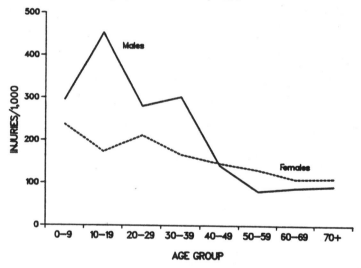

Falls (25.2%) were the most frequent cause of ER visits, followed by sports-related injuries (14.0%) and unintentional cutting/piercing injuries (13.1%) (Table 1). Motor vehicles were involved in 56.9% of the 144 vehicle-related injuries; bicycles were involved in 30.6%; and motorcycles, in 5.5%. The highest rates for all injuries occurred during the late summer and early fall.

The category, "other unintentional injuries," included 12 poisonings, nine of which involved children less than 4 years of age. Three of these children had consumed

---

*Analysis based on 1984 population of the Eastern Band of the Cherokee Indians (6,089).

gasoline, and three had consumed household cleaning agents. Cutting wood with an axe resulted in 11 injuries. Four injuries (including one death) involved firearms.

Most (1,389, or 95.9%) of the injured persons were treated and released. Fifty-one (3.5%) had serious injuries—49 of these were admitted to a local hospital or transferred to a referral hospital, and two died. Eight (0.6%) of the outcomes were unknown. Over half (58.5%) of the patients who were treated and released had lacerations, punctures, contusions, or abrasions. Thirteen (25.5%) of the seriously injured patients had fractures; 12 (23.5%) had lacerations; 7 (13.7%), contusions; 6 (11.8%), head/skull injuries; and 13 (25.5%), other injuries. One-third of the serious injuries were intentional (assaults, stabbings, and gunshot wounds); 23.5% were vehicle-related; and 23.5% were due to falls. Less than 3.0% of the patients with lacerations, punctures, and contusions required hospitalization, whereas 20.0% of those with head/skull injuries and 11.0% of those with fractures required hospitalization. Forty-six percent of those admitted to a hospital required more than 1 day of care. One of the two deaths resulted from a motor vehicle crash, and the other, from a gunshot wound.

TABLE 1. Disposition of injured patients, by type of injury — Cherokee Indian Hospital, Cherokee, North Carolina, July 1, 1984–June 30, 1985

| Type of Injury | Disposition | | | | | | | | | |
| | Treated & Released | | Admitted or Referred | | Died | | Unknown | | Total | |
	No.	(%)	No.	(%)	No.	(%)	No.	(%)	No.	(%)
Unintentional										
Falls	365	(25.2)	12	(0.8)	0	—	1	(0.1)	378	**(26.1)**
Sports-Related	202	(14.0)	0	—	0	—	3	(0.2)	205	**(14.2)**
Cutting/Piercing	190	(13.1)	4	(0.3)	0	—	0	—	194	**(13.4)**
Vehicular	132	(9.1)	11	(0.8)	1	(0.1)	0	—	144	**(9.9)**
Machinery	105	(7.3)	3	(0.2)	0	—	0	—	108	**(7.5)**
Animal-Related	35	(2.4)	0	—	0	—	1	(0.1)	36	**(2.5)**
Fire	6	(0.4)	0	—	0	—	1	(0.1)	7	**(0.5)**
Other	173	(11.9)	2	(0.1)	0	—	0	—	175	**(12.1)**
Intentional	152	(10.5)	16	(1.1)	1	(0.1)	2	(0.1)	171	**(11.8)**
Unknown	29	(2.0)	1	(0.1)	0	—	0	—	30	**(2.1)**
Total	**1,389**	**(95.9)**	**49**	**(3.4)**	**2**	**(0.1)**	**8**	**(0.6)**	**1,448**	**(~100.0)**

Reported by: J Moore, J Mills, Cherokee Svc Unit, Indian Health Svc (IHS), Cherokee, North Carolina. J Meredith, Nashville Area IHS, Nashville, Tennessee. RJ Smith III, Environmental Health Br, IHS, Rockville, Maryland. HJ Winick, MPH, Univ of Minnesota School of Public Health, Minneapolis. Div of Injury Epidemiology and Control, Center for Environmental Health and Injury Control, CDC.

Editorial Note: The combined unintentional and intentional injury mortality rate among the American Indian/Alaskan Native population is three times the rate for the general U.S. population (1). Injuries account for more than 12.0% of all hospitalizations in Indian Health Service (IHS) hospitals and over 5.0% of the outpatient visits at IHS clinics (2).

ER records offer a unique opportunity to develop population-based surveillance for injuries. One limitation of ER-based surveillance, however, is that it does not include data on injuries resulting in death at the scene. Data analyzed in this study noted two deaths. However, during the same period, the North Carolina Medical Examiner received reports on five injury-related deaths involving American Indians residing in the five counties of the Cherokee Indian Reservation.

This study indicated that the most serious injuries occurring in the Cherokee Service Unit are intentional injuries, vehicle-related injuries, and falls. As a result of these findings, the tribal council, the Community Injury Control Committee, and other community leaders and organizations have planned interventions to decrease sports-related injuries, improve roads, and reduce intentional injuries. In addition, activities encouraging the use of seat belts and child-restraint seats to reduce vehicle-related injuries have been planned.

The IHS, working with the tribes, the Bureau of Indian Affairs, and other community groups, coordinates a variety of injury prevention activities including health fairs, national poster and essay contests, and school safety programs. This campaign provides an opportunity for a variety of interested health professionals and organizations to participate in injury prevention programs. To increase the awareness of injuries as a preventable health problem, the IHS designated November as the 5th Annual American Indian/Alaskan Native Safety Awareness Month.

References
1. Indian Health Service. Bridging the gap: report on the task force on parity of Indian health services. Washington, DC: US Department of Health and Human Services, Public Health Service, 1986.
2. Smith SM, Molloy BK, Graitcer PL. Intentional and unintentional injuries at three Indian Health Service units, 1981-1985 [Abstract]. In: Program and abstracts of the 22nd annual meeting of the U.S. Public Health Service Professional Association. Washington, DC: Commissioned Officers Association of the U.S. Public Health Service, 1987.

Update: External Cause-of-Injury Coding in Hospital Discharge Data — United States, 1994

The 1993 national plan for injury prevention and control includes the reporting of E-codes in hospital discharge data whenever injury is the principal diagnosis. Hospital discharge data that include E-codes are useful for establishing state injury-control program priorities; evaluating the etiology of severe injuries; conducting surveillance for childhood injuries; assessing the cost of injuries by external cause; and identifying major causes of home and leisure injuries.

—MMWR Vol. 43/No. 25, July 1, 1994, pp. 465–7

Update: External Cause-of-Injury Coding in Hospital Discharge Data — United States, 1994

Although analysis of hospital discharge data (HDD) can provide important information about severe nonfatal injuries, HDD often do not include information about the causes of these injuries (e.g., motor-vehicle crashes and assaults). Inconsistent reporting of causes of injury has limited the usefulness of HDD for injury surveillance. The *International Classification of Diseases, Ninth Revision, Clinical Modification* (ICD-9-CM) includes codes for classifying external causes of injury (E-codes). This report describes progress in implementing E-code reporting in states.

In June 1991, the National Committee on Vital and Health Statistics (NCVHS) (a legislatively mandated advisory committee of the U.S. Department of Health and Human Services) recommended that E-codes be included in hospital discharge data sets. In addition, because the uniform billing form for hospitals is used frequently as the source for HDD, the NCVHS recommended that the revised uniform billing form (UB-92) designate a space for an E-code (*1*). In February 1992, a UB-92 that included a labeled space for E-codes was approved by the National Uniform Billing Committee (a committee comprising representatives from payor and provider organizations and recognized by the Health Care Financing Administration) for use by all U.S. hospitals (*1*). During October 1993–April 1994, all U.S. hospitals implemented use of the UB-92.

From April 1992 through April 1994, the number of states that required reporting of E-codes in HDD increased from six to 15*. Legislatures in nine of these states enacted laws requiring E-code reporting; six states used another administrative mechanism (e.g., regulations). Two states also required reporting of E-codes for persons treated in outpatient settings (e.g., emergency departments and outpatient clinics). In eight states, the state health department assists institutions in implementing E-code reporting and monitors compliance with reporting requirements; in seven states, other organizations (e.g., organizations that gather state health data) maintain this responsibility.

Reported by: Div of Unintentional Injuries Prevention, National Center for Injury Prevention and Control; Office of Planning and Extramural Programs, National Center for Health Statistics, CDC.

Editorial Note: Because of the importance of collecting information about causes of injury, the 1993 national plan for injury prevention and control includes a recommendation for mandatory reporting of E-codes in HDD whenever injury is the principal diagnosis (*2*). The Council of State and Territorial Epidemiologists, the American Public Health Association, the American Health Information Management Association, the National Association of Health Data Organizations (NAHDA), and other organizations also support the mandatory reporting of E-codes in HDD.

As of April 1994, 27 states had HDD systems that were actively gathering information; in 21 (78%) of these states, the UB-92 was used to collect these data (M. Epstein, NAHDA, personal communication, 1994). The availability of a labeled space for an E-code on the UB-92 has prompted states to collect more consistently these data in HDD.

Reporting of E-codes is useful for establishing priorities for state injury-control programs and for evaluating the etiology of severe injuries—including brain and spinal cord injuries. HDD that include E-codes also are useful in conducting surveillance for

---

*California, Connecticut, Delaware, Maryland, Massachusetts, Missouri, Nebraska, New Jersey, New York, Pennsylvania, Rhode Island, South Carolina, Vermont, Washington, and Wisconsin.

childhood injuries (*3*) and assessing the cost of injuries by external cause (e.g., motorcycle-related injuries) (*4*). To plan, implement, and evaluate injury-prevention programs, states should require the reporting of E-codes in HDD to obtain information about the causes of severe nonfatal injuries (*5*).

CDC is evaluating the ICD-9-CM E-coding system, including the list of E-codes and coding index, and is developing and testing coding guidelines and training materials. Additional information on E-coding is available to state and local health departments from CDC's National Center for Injury Prevention and Control, telephone (404) 488-4652.

References
1. CDC. External cause-of-injury coding in hospital discharge data—United States, 1992. MMWR 1992;41:249–51.
2. CDC. Injury control in the 1990's: a national plan for action. Atlanta: US Department of Health and Human Services, Public Health Service, CDC, National Center for Injury Prevention and Control, 1993.
3. Gallagher SS, Finison K, Guyer B, Goodenough S. The incidence of injuries among 87,000 Massachusetts children and adolescents: results of the 1980–81 statewide Childhood Injury Prevention Program Surveillance System. Am J Public Health 1984;74:1340–7.
4. Rivara FP, Morgan P, Bergman AB, Maier RV. Cost estimates for statewide reporting of injuries by E coding hospital discharge abstract data base systems. Public Health Rep 1990;105:635–6.
5. Sniezek JE, Finklea JF, Graitcer PL. Injury coding and hospital discharge data. JAMA 1989; 262:2270–2.

Economic Impact

Medical-Care Spending — United States

The data in this report corroborate the finding that medical-care payments for injury are the second leading source of direct medical costs in the noninstitutionalized U.S. population. Because direct medical costs do not include reduced or lost productivity in the working-age population, this analysis does not adequately present the total economic burden attributable to injury.

—MMWR Vol. 43/No. 32, August 19, 1994, pp. 581–6

Medical-Care Spending — United States

One aspect of health-care reform is the role of prevention in controlling costs. To evaluate data on medical spending by disease category, the National Public Services Research Institute examined data from the 1987 National Medical Expenditure Survey (NMES-2), with emphasis on the Medical Provider Survey supplement. This report presents the findings of that analysis.

The NMES-2 was a population-based longitudinal survey in which data were gathered for the civilian, noninstitutionalized U.S. population for January 1–December 31, 1987 (the most recent year for which complete data were available), about socio-demographic factors; use of medical care; and medical-care expenditures for hospital inpatient, outpatient, and emergency department care; physician and allied health professional services; prescribed medication; emergency transport; and medical supplies and equipment (1). The Medical Provider Survey supplement provided con-

TABLE 1. Medical expenditures, by diagnostic category,* — United States, 1987[†]

Diagnostic category	Medical expenditures[§]	% Total costs[¶]
Cardiovascular	$ 79.6	13.9
Injury and long-term effects	69.1	12.1
Neoplasm	49.6	8.7
Genitourinary	49.3	8.7
Pregnancy/Birth-related	39.7	6.9
Respiratory	38.3	6.7
Digestive	35.9	6.3
Musculoskeletal**	27.7	4.8
Other circulatory diagnosis	20.2	3.5
Mental health[††]	19.3	3.4
Well care	17.4	3.0
Congenital anomalies	8.7	1.5
Medical misadventure	6.9	1.2
Miscellaneous[§§]	110.6	19.3
Total	**572.3**	**100.0**

*International Classification of Diseases, Ninth Revision, Clinical Modification (ICD-9-CM) codes used to define diagnostic categories: Cardiovascular: 390–429, 451–459; Injury and long-term effects: 800–994, 294.0, 304.6, 310.2, 344.0, 344.1, 366.2, 507.1, 508.0, 521.2, 525.1, 719.0, 719.5, 722.0–722.2, 724.2, 724.3, 724.5, 724.6, 724.8, 780.0, 799.0, V71.3–V71.5; Neoplasms: 140–239, V58.0, V58.1; Genitourinary: 580–629, 250.0, V56; Pregnancy and birth-related conditions, including live births and normal delivery: 630–674, V22.2; Respiratory: 460–519, 786.0 (excluding codes used for the injury diagnostic category); Digestive: 520–579 (excluding codes used for the injury diagnostic category); Musculoskeletal: 710–739 (excluding codes used for the injury diagnostic category); Other circulatory: 430–450; Mental disease: 290–319 (excluding codes used for the injury diagnostic category); Well care: V40–V49, V70–V82 (excluding codes used for the injury diagnostic category); Congenital anomalies: 740–779; Medical misadventure: 995–999; and Miscellaneous: all other ICD-9-CM codes.
[†]Adjusted to December 1993 dollars. Excludes nursing home, dental, and insurance claims processing costs.
[§]In billions.
[¶]Costs of incidents without diagnoses were allocated in proportion to cost of known diagnoses.
**Musculoskeletal problems traceable to earlier injury were classified as injury.
[††]Excludes mental health services without a medical component.
[§§]Miscellaneous includes carpal tunnel syndrome, endocrine disorders other than diabetes, anemia, conditions that were not clearly attributable to an underlying cause (e.g., unconsciousness, headache, and fitting and adjustment of prostheses), cataracts, and glaucoma.

firmation of self-reported medical-care costs and information about costs that survey respondents were unable to report. The analysis presented in this report was restricted to the household survey sample of the NMES-2, a subset of the data that included face-to-face interviews of approximately 35,000 persons in 14,000 households regarding use of and expenses for health services during 1987. Not included in this analysis were dental costs, mental health services without a medical component, and administrative costs and overhead for insurance claims. All medical expenditure estimates were adjusted to December 1993 dollars using medical-care spending per capita for all medical treatment as the inflator.

Cardiovascular disease accounted for $80 billion (14%) of the $572 billion (in 1993 dollars) in medical spending for services other than nursing-home care, dental care, and insurance claims processing (Table 1). Injuries accounted for $69 billion (12%), including spending attributed to longer term musculoskeletal deterioration resulting from injury. Spending for each of these categories exceeded that for cancer and for genitourinary disease (including kidney disease) ($49 billion each). Medical spending for well care, including preventive care, was 3% of the total costs ($17 billion).

Excluding live births, injury was the largest contributor to health-care expenditures for persons aged 5–49 years (Figure 1). Injury was the second largest contributor to health-care costs among persons aged <5 years and >85 years; cardiovascular disease and cancer were the two largest contributors for those aged 50–85 years.

Medical spending on injury treatment averaged $284 per person. Injury costs increased for those aged >65 years, with the highest per capita spending for injury being

FIGURE 1. Percentage of medical-care spending, by age group and selected causes — National Medical Expenditures Survey, United States, 1987*

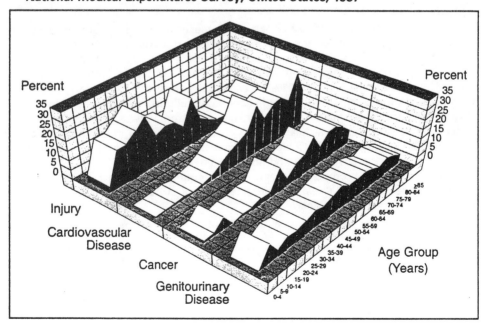

*Excludes nursing home, dental, and insurance claims processing costs.

FIGURE 2. Injury cost per person, by age group — National Medical Expenditure Survey, United States, 1987*

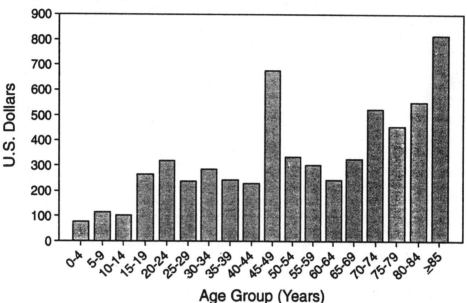

*Adjusted to December 1993 dollars. Excludes nursing home, dental, and insurance claims processing costs.

for those aged ≥70 years (Figure 2). However, increases in spending for cardiovascular disease and cancer for those age groups were higher than those for injury.

Inpatient hospital costs were the largest component of medical spending ($329 billion [57%]), with ambulatory-care visits contributing $90 billion (16%) and hospital outpatient services, $66 billion (11%). Prescriptions were the fourth largest component ($38 billion [7%]). Home-health–care ($20 billion), emergency department ($15 billion), and other medical ($15 billion) costs each contributed approximately 3%.

By type of care, cardiovascular disease accounted for 15% of the hospital costs; cancer, 11%; and injury, 10% (Table 2). Cardiovascular disease also contributed the most in prescription costs (27%) and home-health–care costs (27%) (Table 2). Injury costs were the largest component of spending for emergency department visits (46%), hospital outpatient visits (16%), and ambulatory care (16%). Of the ambulatory-care visit costs, 14% were for well care.

Reported by: TR Miller, PhD, DC Lestina, MS Galbraith, Children's Safety Network Economics and Insurance Resource Center, National Public Svcs Research Institute, Landover, Maryland. DC Viano, PhD, Biomedical Science Dept, General Motors Research Laboratories, Warren, Michigan. Div of Unintentional Injury Prevention, National Center for Injury Prevention and Control, CDC.

TABLE 2. Percentage of expenditures for different types of care, by diagnostic category* — United States, 1987[†]

Diagnostic category	Hospital inpatient care	Emergency department	Outpatient care	Ambulatory visits	Home care	Prescriptions	Other
Cardiovascular	15.1	4.6	9.6	7.3	27.3	27.1	3.5
Injury and long-term effects	10.1	45.9	16.1	16.4	7.3	3.4	7.7
Neoplasm	10.7	10.2	11.3	4.4	7.7	3.0	1.8
Genitourinary	8.8	5.7	12.6	6.4	10.4	7.5	4.9
Pregnancy/ Birth-related	10.2	1.2	0.5	4.1	0.0	0.2	0.1
Respiratory	6.2	10.7	6.2	7.7	3.0	10.5	5.0
Digestive	8.4	4.4	4.2	2.8	1.0	4.9	0.8
Musculoskeletal[§]	3.3	2.7	7.8	6.4	11.9	7.3	3.5
Other circulatory	5.1	0.9	1.2	1.0	3.4	1.6	0.9
Mental health[¶]	3.2	1.2	2.6	5.5	3.1	3.8	0.1
Well care	0.1	<0.1	1.5	13.6	1.8	1.4	1.0
Congenital anomalies	2.1	0.2	1.0	0.5	0.3	1.2	0.4
Medical misadventure	1.3	2.1	1.4	1.0	0.3	1.1	0.5
Miscellaneous**	14.5	18.8	24.1	22.9	22.5	27.0	69.8
Total	**100.0**	**100.0**	**100.0**	**100.0**	**100.0**	**100.0**	**100.0**

* *International Classification of Diseases, Ninth Revision, Clinical Modification* (ICD-9-CM) codes used to define diagnostic categories: Cardiovascular: 390–429, 451–459; Injury and long-term effects: 800–994, 294.0, 304.6, 310.2, 344.0, 344.1, 366.2, 507.1, 508.0, 521.2, 525.1, 719.0, 719.5, 722.0–722.2, 724.2, 724.3, 724.5, 724.6, 724.8, 780.0, 799.0, V71.3–V71.5; Neoplasms: 140–239, V58.0, V58.1; Genitourinary: 580–629, 250.0, V56; Pregnancy and birth-related conditions, including live births and normal delivery: 630–674, V22.2; Respiratory: 460–519, 786.0 (excluding codes used for the injury diagnostic category); Digestive: 520–579 (excluding codes used for the injury diagnostic category); Musculoskeletal: 710–739 (excluding codes used for the injury diagnostic category); Other circulatory: 430–450; Mental disease: 290–319 (excluding codes used for the injury diagnostic category); Well care: V40–V49, V70–V82 (excluding codes used for the injury diagnostic category); Congenital anomalies: 740–779; Medical misadventure: 995–999; and Miscellaneous: all other ICD-9-CM codes.
[†] Adjusted to December 1993 dollars. Excludes nursing home, dental, and insurance claims processing costs.
[§] Musculoskeletal problems traceable to earlier injury were classified as injury.
[¶] Excludes mental health services without a medical component.
** Miscellaneous includes carpal tunnel syndrome, endocrine disorders other than diabetes, anemia, conditions that were not clearly attributable to an underlying cause (e.g., unconsciousness, headache, and fitting and adjustment of prostheses), cataracts, and glaucoma.

Editorial Note: The findings in this report indicate that the largest source of health-care spending in the U.S. population is cardiovascular disease. This reflects the high prevalence of coronary or ischemic heart disease, which is the leading cause of death in the United States. However, the influences and risk factors for cardiovascular disease potentially can be modified through public policy and preventive practice (e.g., smoking and diet).

Injury, the leading cause of death for persons in all age groups from 1 year through 44 years (2), is also a large contributor to health-care costs. The data in this report corroborate the finding that medical-care payments for injury are the second leading source of direct medical costs in the noninstitutionalized U.S. population (3). In addition, the cost burden for injuries is spread across all age groups (4). Because direct medical costs do not include the reduced or lost productivity in the working-age population, this analysis does not adequately present the total economic burden attributable to injury.

This study is subject to at least four limitations. First, the data underestimate total direct medical costs because institutionalized persons, military members and their families, and homeless persons were excluded. Second, nursing home costs—approximately $60 billion annually across all disease categories (5)—also were omitted from this analysis. Third, the unitary, systems-based categorization of each illness or injury used in this analysis masks the potential importance of some categories, such as infectious diseases. Infectious diseases were subsumed under the injury or system category that they affect; for example, pulmonary infections tended to be classified in the respiratory category, urinary tract infections in the genitourinary category, and human immunodeficiency virus (HIV) infection and acquired immunodeficiency syndrome (AIDS) in the categories of affected systems or as miscellaneous. Similarly, spending for outpatient visits for complications of diabetes mellitus may appear as cardiovascular disease costs. Fourth, the direct costs related to infectious diseases are underestimated because the incidence of HIV infection and AIDS resulted in substantially increased spending after 1987 (6).

Numerous prevention measures reduce direct medical costs while saving lives. For example, approximately $2 are saved in medical-care costs for every $1 spent on child-safety seats (7); from 1982 through 1990, child-safety seats and safety belts saved the lives of approximately 1300 infants and toddlers in the United States (8). The data in this report underscore the impact of different disease categories and the need to evaluate the relative effectiveness and the cost-effectiveness of interventions that prevent and control the effects of disease; such data can assist in making decisions regarding treatment and prevention programs (9).

References
1. Edwards WS, Berlin M. Questionnaires and data collection methods for the household survey and the survey of American Indians and Alaskan Natives. Rockville, Maryland: US Department of Health and Human Services, Public Health Service, National Center for Health Services Research and Health Care Technology Assessment, 1989; DHHS publication no. (PHS)89-3450. (National Medical Expenditure Survey Methods 2.)
2. NCHS. Health, United States, 1992. Washington, DC: US Department of Health and Human Services, Public Health Service, CDC, 1993; DHHS publication no. (PHS)93-1232.
3. Harlan LC, Harlan WR, Parsons PE. The economic impact of injuries: a major source of medical costs. Am J Public Health 1990;80:453–9.
4. Max W, Rice DP, MacKenzie EJ. The lifetime cost of injury. Inquiry 1990;27:332–43.
5. Bureau of the Census. Statistical abstract of the United States, 1993. Washington, DC: US Department of Commerce, Bureau of the Census, 1993.
6. Mann JM, Tarantola DJM, Netter TW, eds. AIDS in the world. Cambridge, Massachusetts: Harvard University Press, 1992:316.
7. Miller TR, Demes JC, Bovbjerg RR. Child seats: how large are the benefits and who should pay? In: Child occupant protection [Monograph]. Warrendale, Pennsylvania: Society of Automotive Engineers 1993:81–9; publication no. SP-986.
8. National Highway Traffic Safety Administration. Occupant protection facts. Washington, DC: US Department of Transportation, National Highway Traffic Safety Administration, 1990.
9. Public Health Service/Battelle. For a healthy nation: returns on investment in public health. Atlanta: US Department of Health and Human Services, Public Health Service, Office of Disease Prevention and Health Promotion and CDC/Battelle, Center for Public Health Research and Evaluation, 1994.

Falls

Deaths from Falls, 1978–1984

Overall, fall-related mortality rates are declining in the United States. The crude annual rate of deaths per 100,000 persons declined from 6.2 in 1978 to 5.1 in 1984. Unfortunately, much useful information about the place and type of fall is often unavailable. To reduce morbidity and mortality caused by falls, public health personnel need more information about the effectiveness of interventions and the circumstances and risk factors for falls and fall-related injuries.

—MMWR Vol. 37/No. SS-1, February 1988, pp. 21–6

Deaths from Falls, 1978–1984

Deborah A. Lambert, R.N., M.S.
Richard W. Sattin, M.D.
Division of Injury Epidemiology and Control
Center for Environmental Health and Injury Control

Introduction

Falls are the leading cause of nonfatal injury and the second leading cause of unintentional injury-related deaths in the United States, surpassed only by motor vehicle-related deaths (*1-3*). Falls cause more deaths per year than drownings and fires combined (*2*). Although the cost of falls in the United States is not known, injuries cost this country between $75 billion and $100 billion each year in direct and indirect costs (*3*).

As a result of the Surgeon General's report in 1979 titled "Healthy People," which indicated that many deaths and injuries due to falls were preventable, a measurable objective of no more than two deaths per 100,000 persons by the year 1990 was established (*4,5*). This report 1) describes the epidemiology of falls in the United States, 2) reviews the progress made since 1978 toward meeting the 1990 objective, 3) discusses factors that may have either improved or hindered this progress, and 4) recommends ways to reduce fall-related mortality.

Methods

For this report, the number of deaths from falls for the years 1978-1984 were determined by using data from annual mortality tapes compiled by the National Center for Health Statistics (NCHS). The NCHS receives vital statistics on deaths from all 50 states and the District of Columbia. For this report, only U.S. residents who died in the United States are included. Information available from the NCHS mortality tapes includes age, sex, race (white, black, other), state of decedent's residence, state in which death occurred, and date of death.

For 1978, fall-related deaths were defined as those with an external underlying cause of death coded as E880 to E887 according to the International Classification of Diseases (ICD), Adapted, Eighth Revision. For the years 1979-1984, fall-related deaths were defined as those with an external underlying cause of death coded as E880 to E888 according to the ICD, Ninth Revision. Regions of the country (Northeast, Midwest, South, and West) were defined according to NCHS guidelines. Place where the fall occurred was defined according to NCHS and ICD criteria as home, farm, mine and quarry, industrial place and premises, place for recreation and sport, street and highway, public building, residential institution, other specified places, or place of occurrence not specified.

The population data used in computing crude death rates per 100,000 population were obtained from the Bureau of the Census. For 1980, the census enumeration of the population was used, and for 1978-1979 and 1981-1984, population estimates from the Bureau of the Census were used. Regional rates were based on deaths of residents of the respective regions.

Results

The number of deaths from falls declined from 13,690 in 1978 to 11,937 in 1984 (Table 1). The annual death rate from falls for the same period dropped from 6.2 to

5.1/100,000 persons. During the 7-year period, the percent declines in the total number of fall deaths and in the fall death rate were 12.8 and 17.7, respectively. For each of the four age groups, the overall death rate declined 18%-26% from 1978 through 1984. A slight increase in rate occurred in 1984 among persons ages 65-84 years. In 1984, the ratio of fall-related death rates for persons ages ≥85 years was 98.0 when compared with those <65 years, 14.4 when compared with those ages 65-74 years, and 4.0 when compared with those ages 75-84 years.

More males than females died from falls each year (Table 1). Regardless of sex, both the number and the rate of fall-related deaths declined overall. For males, however, the number of deaths and the death rate rose slightly in 1980; for females, the number of deaths, but not the death rate, rose slightly in 1983. The ratio of fall-related death rates for males compared with females was 1.2 for each of the years 1978-1982 and for 1984, and it was 1.1 for 1983.

Overall, all races had declines in both the number of deaths and the death rate from falls (Table 1). In 1980, however, the number of deaths for whites and blacks did increase slightly, and both the number and rate increased for other races. In 1984, the number but not the rate of fall-related deaths increased slightly for other races. Whites consistently had the highest death rates from falls, whereas other races had the lowest. Compared with other races, whites had a 2.7-fold increased rate, and blacks had a 1.8-fold increased rate in 1984.

Regional rates also varied (Table 1). The Northeast, the region with the highest fall-related death rate for each of the years, had a decline in rates over the entire

TABLE 1. Deaths due to falls, by characteristics and year, United States, 1978-1984

Characteristic	1978 No.	1978 Rate*	1979 No.	1979 Rate	1980 No.	1980 Rate	1981 No.	1981 Rate	1982 No.	1982 Rate	1983 No.	1983 Rate	1984 No.	1984 Rate*
Age group (years)†														
<65	4,008	2.0	3,801	1.9	3,941	2.0	3,601	1.8	3,448	1.7	3,367	1.6	3,168	1.5
65-74	1,852	12.4	1,956	12.8	1,840	11.8	1,721	10.8	1,635	10.1	1,656	10.1	1,702	10.2
75-84	3,715	50.1	3,612	47.5	3,482	44.7	3,313	41.4	3,232	39.2	3,113	36.5	3,204	37.2
85+	4,109	196.2	3,844	175.0	4,026	177.3	3,985	169.5	3,757	154.2	3,880	155.0	3,857	147.0
Sex														
Male	7,181	6.7	6,928	6.3	7,036	6.4	6,627	5.9	6,354	5.6	6,279	5.5	6,210	5.5
Female	6,509	5.7	6,288	5.4	6,258	5.4	6,001	5.1	5,723	4.8	5,745	4.8	5,727	4.7
Race														
White	12,405	6.5	11,999	6.2	12,016	6.2	11,417	5.8	10,930	5.5	10,877	5.5	10,829	5.4
Black	1,145	4.4	1,110	4.2	1,124	4.2	1,074	3.9	1,027	3.7	1,018	3.6	976	3.5
Other	140	3.3	107	2.4	154	2.9	137	2.4	120	2.0	129	2.0	132	2.0
Region														
Northeast	3,373	6.9	3,281	6.7	3,192	6.5	2,907	5.9	2,918	5.9	2,909	5.9	2,790	5.7
Midwest	3,911	6.7	3,736	6.4	3,632	6.2	3,480	5.9	3,282	5.6	3,404	5.8	3,202	5.4
South	4,151	5.7	4,009	5.4	4,093	5.4	3,984	5.2	3,747	4.8	3,602	4.6	3,662	4.7
West	2,255	5.5	2,190	5.2	2,377	5.5	2,257	5.2	2,130	4.8	2,109	4.6	2,283	5.0
Total	13,690	6.2	13,216	5.9	13,294	5.9	12,628	5.5	12,077	5.2	12,024	5.1	11,937	5.1

*Deaths/100,000 persons.
†Number of deaths may not reflect total because in some instances the decedent's age was unknown.

period. In 1984, that region's death rate from falls was about 1.2 times that for the South, the region with the lowest rate. The trend in the Midwest, the region with the second highest fall-related death rate, was similar to that for the Northeast except for a slight increase in rate in 1983. Despite a 1980 increase in the West and a 1984 increase in the West and South in fall-related mortality rates, the West and South—regions with the lowest death rates—had overall declines in fall-related death rates in the period 1978-1984.

White males ages ≥85 years had the highest age-, sex-, race-specific death rate of 187.2/100,000 persons in 1984 (Figure 1). For persons ages 5-29 years and ages ≥75 years, white males had the highest fall-related death rate. Males of all other races had the highest rate among persons <5 years and those ages 30-69 years. Females of all other races had higher death rates than white females until the age of 65 years, the only exceptions being the 10- to 24- and the 50- to 54-year age groups. After age 65, females of all other races had the lowest race- and sex-specific death rate from falls. After age 75, the death rate for white females exceeded that for males and females of all other races.

FIGURE 1. Rate of fall-related deaths, by age group, race, and sex, United States, 1984

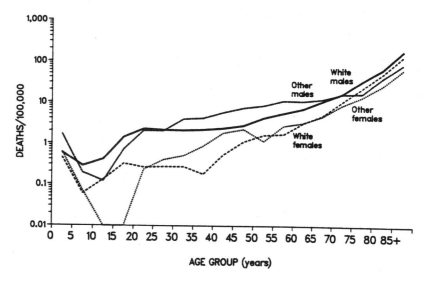

The largest proportion of fall-related deaths occurred in the winter and autumn (Table 2). However, the percentage of deaths both overall and by region did not vary considerably or consistently by season.

In about one-fourth (3,299) of the fall-related deaths, the place where the fall occurred was not specified on the death certificate (Table 3). In 1984, over 43% of the deaths (5,166) occurred in the home. Almost 67% of children <5 years old who died from a fall died in the home. Of all persons ≥65 years of age who died from falls, about 45% died from a fall in the home and about 15% from a fall in a residential institution.

TABLE 2. Number and percentage of fall-related deaths, by time of year and region of residence, United States, 1984

Months	Northeast No.	(%)*	Midwest No.	(%)	South No.	(%)	West No.	(%)	Total No.	(%)
Dec-Feb	725	(26.0)	793	(24.8)	927	(25.3)	600	(26.3)	3,045	(25.5)
Mar-May	688	(24.7)	814	(25.4)	925	(25.3)	520	(22.8)	2,947	(24.7)
Jun-Aug	649	(23.3)	780	(24.4)	895	(24.4)	581	(25.4)	2,905	(24.3)
Sep-Nov	728	(26.1)	815	(25.5)	915	(25.0)	582	(25.5)	3,040	(25.5)
Total	2,790	(100.0)	3,202	(100.0)	3,662	(100.0)	2,283	(100.0)	11,937	(100.0)

*Percentages may not total 100.0 because of rounding.

TABLE 3. Number of fall-related deaths, by age group and place where fall occurred, United States, 1984

Age group (years)*	Home	Residential institution	Other specified	Unknown	Total
<5	76	1	16	21	114
5-9	9	0	12	6	27
10-19	17	4	149	17	187
20-44	315	38	710	153	1,216
45-64	798	87	491	248	1,624
≥65	3,951	1,356	602	2,854	8,763
Total	5,166	1,486	1,980	3,299	11,931

*Six deaths were excluded because decedent's age was unknown.

Discussion

In this study of deaths caused by falls, the results show that the crude annual death rate/100,000 persons declined from 6.2 in 1978 to 5.1 in 1984. Children of races other than white, especially males <5 years old, males of races other than white ages 30-69 years, and white males ≥70 years of age were among those with the highest death rates. The Northeast had the highest regional rate, and the South had the lowest. Most children <5 years of age and many elderly persons who died from falls had fallen at home.

Several limitations may have affected the estimated fall-related death rates in this report. First, the rates may have been underestimated because falls are under-reported as the underlying cause of death (1). No data exist to show if this underreporting changed between 1978 and 1984. Second, death rates from falls may have been overestimated for blacks, who were underenumerated in the 1980 census (6). However, adjusting the rates found in this study by the proposed underenumeration did not appreciably alter the findings.

Unfortunately, much useful information about the place and type of the fall is often unavailable. For example, in about one-fourth of the deaths in this study, the death certificate did not show the place of occurrence. Moreover, about 46% of fall-related deaths were coded as E888 (other and unknown), and about 22% were coded as E887 (fracture with unspecified cause), thus precluding a useful analysis by the type of fall.

As people age, the risk of death from a fall increases. People ≥85 years of age are at the greatest risk of death from a fall. Impairments such as poor vision, unsteady gait, and chronic medical conditions may predispose an individual to fall or may contribute to the death once a fall occurs (1). Environmental factors, such as stairway design and disrepair, inadequate lighting, and slipping and tripping on water, ice, clutter, loose rugs, or electrical cords, may also play a key role in the occurrence of a fall (1,7).

During their middle-aged years, males are at greater risk than females of dying from a fall. The larger number of men working in hazardous occupations, such as construction, may increase their risk of falling from heights and sustaining more severe injuries than females. Why black males have an increased risk of dying from falls during the middle-aged years is unclear and needs further study.

Black children are at a greater risk of death from falls than white children. Several reasons for this finding might include a higher percentage of blacks living in substandard high-rise buildings (8), less ability of the poor to provide constant supervision for their children, and delayed emergency response time in rural areas.

The higher fall-related death rates in the Northeast and Midwest compared with those in the South and West might be explained by differences in the climate, the level of urbanization, and the age and racial distribution in the four regions. For example, the Northeast has more inclement weather, more urban areas, more whites, and a larger older population than the South. The percentage of fall-related deaths by season, however, did not appreciably differ in any of the regions.

Overall, fall-related mortality rates are declining in the United States. The reason is unclear, but the decline may be due to improved medical care and services (1). Several interventions may have helped to reduce the number of deaths due to falls, although few have been evaluated for their effectiveness (1,7-10). In New York City, after a law was passed requiring landlords to provide window guards in apartments where young children live, the number of falls dropped significantly (9). Improved lighting and handrail installation and use have also been suggested to reduce the incidence of falls (1,7,10). In addition, increased dietary intake of calcium and estrogen replacement therapy for postmenopausal women are believed to delay or reduce osteoporosis, thus reducing injuries that result from falls (10).

To reduce morbidity and mortality caused by falls, public health personnel need more information about the effectiveness of interventions and the contributing factors to the risk of falling and sustaining an injury. More complete information is also needed about the circumstances of falls that result in injury or death.

The 1990 objective has limited usefulness as an indicator of the public health impact of fall-related mortality. The objective is based on an overall crude death rate and does not focus on specific high-risk groups. For example, elderly persons account for an increasing percentage of the population; therefore, the overall crude death rate from falls may increase in the future because of high death rates in this group. Future objectives for the nation related to falls should focus on morbidity and mortality in high-risk populations.

Given the current rate of decline, the death rate due to falls would be 4.2/100,000 persons in 1990, far short of the 1990 target of 2.0/100,000 persons (Figure 2). If fall-related injuries and deaths are to be substantially reduced, efforts should focus on determining risk factors for falls, determining which risk factors can be prevented or ameliorated, and evaluating the effectiveness of the prevention measures in reducing morbidity, severity, and mortality. Furthermore, the public health impact of falls cannot be fully understood without assessing the incidence of nonfatal injuries from falls. To close this gap in knowledge, national surveys that now collect data on the anatomic nature (N codes) of injuries due to falls should also collect information on the external cause (E codes) of these injuries.

FIGURE 2. Death rates from falls, by year, United States, 1978-1984

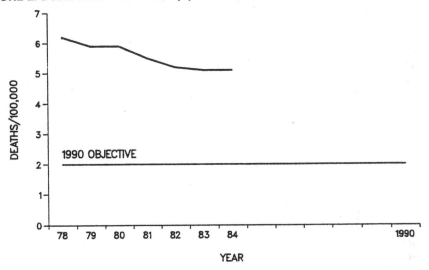

References
1. Baker SP, O'Neill B, Karpf RS. The injury fact book. Lexington, Massachusetts: Lexington Books, DC Heath and Company, 1984.
2. National Safety Council. Accident facts. Chicago: National Safety Council, 1985.
3. Committee on Trauma Research, Commission on Life Sciences, National Research Council, and the Institute on Medicine. Injury in America. Washington, DC: National Academy Press, 1985.
4. US Department of Health, Education, and Welfare, Public Health Service. Healthy people: the Surgeon General's report on health promotion and disease prevention. Washington, DC: US Department of Health, Education, and Welfare, 1979; DHEW (PHS) publication no. 79-55071.
5. US Department of Health and Human Services, Public Health Service. Promoting health/ preventing disease: objectives for the nation. Washington, DC: US Department of Health and Human Services, 1980.
6. Savage IR. Who counts? Am Stat 1982;36:195-200.
7. Archea JC. Environmental factors associated with stair accidents by the elderly. Clin Geriatr Med 1985;1(August):555-69.
8. Garrettson LK, Gallagher SS. Falls in children and youth. Pediatr Clin North Am 1985;32:153-62.
9. Spiegel CN, Lindaman FC. Children can't fly: a program to prevent childhood morbidity and mortality from window falls. Am J Public Health 1977;67:1143-7.
10. Hogue CC. Injury in late life: II. Prevention. Am Geriatr Soc 1982;30(April):276-80.

Fires and Burns

Deaths Resulting from Residential Fires — United States, 1991

Residential-fire death rates decreased 37% from 1970 through 1991 but did not achieve the national health objective for the year 2000. Death rates are highest among children <5 years of age and persons ≥65 years of age. To reduce the risk for death or injury from fires, a smoke detector should be installed outside each sleeping area on every habitable level of a home, and the battery should be changed at least annually.

—MMWR Vol. 43/No. 49, December 16, 1994, pp. 901–4

Deaths Resulting from Residential Fires — United States, 1991

Most residential fires occur during December through March—a period of colder weather and longer darkness. During 1991, residential fires were the second leading cause of injury deaths (after motor-vehicle–related injuries) among children aged 1–9 years (*1*) and the sixth leading cause of such deaths among persons aged ≥65 years. Because of seasonal variations in the occurrence of residential fires, CDC analyzed death certificate data from U.S. vital statistics mortality tapes maintained by CDC's National Center for Health Statistics and data from the National Fire Incidence Reporting System (NFIRS) to improve characterization of selected residential fires. This report summarizes the analysis of death certificate data for 1991 and data from NFIRS for 1990.

Deaths from residential fires were identified using *International Classification of Diseases, Ninth Revision*, external cause of injury codes E890–E899 and place of occurrence noted as residence on the death certificate. Information about the causes of fire-associated deaths was obtained from NFIRS, maintained by the U.S. Fire Administration, which gathers detailed reports of a sample of fire-associated deaths collected from approximately 13,500 fire departments in 41 states (*2*). NFIRS estimates of deaths associated with residential fires for children aged <5 years were based on 279 deaths, and for adults aged >70 years, 368 deaths.

In 1991, residential fires accounted for 3683 deaths; of these, 1773 (48%) occurred during January (495), February (415), March (409), and December (454) (Figure 1). These deaths included 711 (19%) among children aged <5 years and 898 (24%) among persons aged ≥70 years. In comparison with the total population, the rate for fire-related death was highest for the young and the elderly (Figure 2).

Based on NFIRS data for January–December 1990, the causes of the fires were known for 522 (72%) deaths of children aged <5 years; the three leading causes were 1) children playing with fire-ignition sources (e.g., matches) (37%), 2) faulty or misused heating devices (19%), and 3) faulty or misused electrical distribution sources* (11%). For persons aged >70 years, the causes of fires were known for 247 (67%) deaths; the three leading causes were 1) careless smoking (33%), 2) faulty or misused heating devices (19%), and 3) faulty or misused electrical distribution sources (12%) (*2*).

Data from the 1990 NFIRS were used to estimate the numbers of fires and deaths associated with selected causes of residential fires during January, February, March, and December (*2*). During these months in 1990, residential electrical-distribution fires were associated with an estimated 40,000 fires and 266 deaths (Table 1). Residential fires involving fireplaces and chimneys resulted in an estimated 26,200 fires, and portable kerosene and electrical heaters were involved in an estimated 1500 fires. Christmas tree fires caused approximately 600 residential fires and 29 deaths; the ratio of deaths to fires was 1:21.

---

*Includes wiring, transformers, meter boxes, power switching gear, outlets, cords, plugs, and lighting fixtures as sources of heat.

FIGURE 1. Number of deaths from residential fires,* by month — United States, 1991

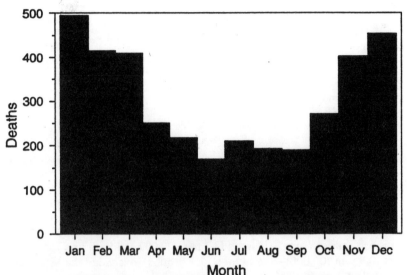

* *International Classification of Diseases, Ninth Revision,* codes E890–E899.

Source: National Center for Health Statistics, CDC.

FIGURE 2. Rate* of deaths from residential fires† during winter months§ and nonwinter months¶, by age group of decedent — United States, 1991

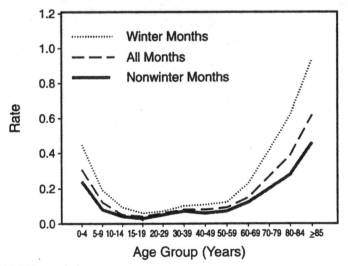

* Per 100,000 population.
† *International Classification of Diseases, Ninth Revision,* codes E890–E899.
§ January, February, March, and December.
¶ April through November.

Source: National Center for Health Statistics, CDC.

TABLE 1. Estimated number of residential fires, number of deaths, and ratio of deaths to fires, by selected causes — United States, 1990

Cause	No. deaths	Estimated no. fires	Ratio (deaths:fires)
Christmas trees	29	600	1:21
Portable heaters	56	1,500	1:27
Electrical distribution*	266	40,000	1:150
Fireplaces and chimneys	58	26,200	1:452

*Includes wiring, transformers, meter boxes, power switching gear, outlets, cords, plugs, and lighting fixtures as sources of heat.

Source: National Fire Incidence Reporting System, U.S. Fire Administration.

Reported by: Div of Unintentional Injury Prevention, National Center for Injury Prevention and Control, CDC.

Editorial Note: Despite the 37% decline in rates of residential-fire deaths from 1970 through 1991 (*1*), the overall rate in 1991 (1.5 per 100,000) exceeded the rate targeted by a national health objective for the year 2000 (reducing the rate of residential fire-related deaths to no more than 1.2 deaths per 100,000 persons [objective 9.6]). In particular, the rates for children aged <5 years (3.7 per 100,000 children) and for persons aged ≥65 years (3.5 per 100,000)—the highest-risk groups—exceeded the age-group–specific target goal of 3.3 per 100,000 for each group (*1,3*).

The increased occurrence of fire-related deaths during winter months reflects the seasonal use of portable heaters, fireplaces and chimneys, and Christmas trees (*2*). Fires associated with electric portable heaters usually result from electrical shortages or device failure, rather than from ignition of nearby materials such as draperies. Electric cords for portable electric space heaters should be plugged directly into the wall and not linked through an extension cord, kept at least 3 feet from any combustible object, and unplugged when not in use. Fires attributed to the use of kerosene portable heaters usually result from using the wrong fuel, faulty switches and valves, and fuel leaks and spills that subsequently ignite. Kerosene heaters should be used only with K-1 kerosene, rather than gasoline or camp-stove fuel, and should be re-fueled outdoors after the heater has cooled. Chimney fires usually result from a build-up of creosote, a highly flammable by-product of wood fires. Chimneys should be cleaned or inspected annually to detect and prevent creosote build-up. A fire screen should be used in front of the fireplace; wood stoves and fireplaces should burn only seasoned wood—not green wood, trash, or wrapping paper.

Fires related to Christmas trees usually result from electrical problems (e.g., overloaded electrical circuits caused by using several extension cords in one outlet, or frayed wire and cords). In 1991, Christmas trees accounted for the lowest number of fires, but a substantially higher proportion of deaths than other types of residential fires described in this report (Table 1). Persons in households with these holiday decorations should periodically examine the electric lights used and should not place trees near heating sources or fireplaces. In addition, live-cut trees should be sufficiently watered to reduce drying; dry trees ignite easily and burn rapidly.

To reduce the risk for death or injury resulting from fires, a smoke detector should be installed outside each sleeping area on every habitable level of a home and the battery changed at least annually. Occupants should develop escape plans that include the identification of two exits from every living area and should practice exit drills and meeting at a designated place at a safe location sufficiently distant from the home. In addition, every home should have a multipurpose fire extinguisher ready for use in extinguishing small fires. Residences should be evacuated for any fire that cannot be extinguished within 1 minute because of the rapid rate of accumulation of heat and smoke; once evacuated, residences should not be reentered. Persons who become trapped in a residence should crawl on the floor toward an exit to avoid inhalation of smoke that has risen.

Because children playing with fire-ignition sources were the leading cause of fires that resulted in the deaths of children aged <5 years, children should be taught not to play with matches or lighters. In addition, young children should be told to inform an adult immediately if they see a fire starting. Other precautions should include storing matches and lighters out of the reach of young children; wooden "strike anywhere" kitchen matches should not be used or kept in homes with young children.

Programs directed at modifying the environment and behaviors may assist in reducing the number of deaths from residential fires. For example, CDC is working with the Maryland Department of Health and Mental Hygiene, Division of Injury and Disability Prevention and Rehabilitation, to install smoke detectors in homes, implement a public health education campaign about smoke detector use and maintenance, and pass and enforce local smoke detector ordinances.

References
1. NCHS. Vital statistics mortality data, underlying cause of death, 1980–1991 [Machine-readable public-use data tapes]. Hyattsville, Maryland: US Department of Health and Human Services, Public Health Service, CDC, NCHS, 1991.
2. Federal Emergency Management Agency. Fire in the United States, 1983–1990. Washington, DC: US Fire Administration, 1993; publication no. USFA/FA-140.
3. Public Health Service. Healthy people 2000: national health promotion and disease prevention objectives—full report, with commentary. Washington, DC: US Department of Health and Human Services, Public Health Service, 1991; DHHS publication no. (PHS)91-50212.

Deaths from Residential Fires, 1978–1984

*Adults aged ≥65 years, children aged <5 years,
and blacks of all ages are at high risk for death
from residential fires. Most deaths from residential fires occur in the winter, and the highest
residential fire-related death rates occur in the
South. Intervention strategies include increasing
ownership of smoke detectors, improving the
flame-retardant property of sleepwear, reducing
the number of people who smoke cigarettes, and
promoting the use of self-extinguishing matches.*

—MMWR Vol. 37/No. SS-1, February 1988, pp. 39–45

Deaths from Residential Fires, 1978–1984

Jama A. Gulaid, Ph.D., M.P.H.
Richard W. Sattin, M.D.
Richard J. Waxweiler, Ph.D.
Division of Injury Epidemiology and Control
Center for Environmental Health and Injury Control

Introduction

Residential fires account for most deaths from fire and flames, the fourth leading cause of injury-related deaths in the United States after motor vehicles, falls, and drownings (*1*). Each year residential fires cause an estimated 19,275 injuries among civilians and involve more than $3.4 billion in property damages (*2*). In 1979, the U.S. Department of Health and Human Services, in its health objectives for 1990, set a specific objective pertaining to residential fires: to reduce the crude death rate due to residential fires from 2.4/100,000 persons in 1978, the baseline year, to 1.5/100,000 persons in 1990 (*3*).

This report provides information on 1) the epidemiology of residential fires in the United States, 2) progress made since 1978 toward the 1990 objective, 3) factors enhancing or impeding progress toward this objective, and 4) recommended measures that will help attain this objective.

Methods

Data used to determine the number of deaths from residential fires for 1978-1984 are from annual mortality tapes of the National Center for Health Statistics (NCHS). NCHS receives reports of all deaths of U.S. residents in the 50 states and the District of Columbia. Deaths are coded according to the International Classification of Diseases (ICD), Adapted—Eighth Revision for 1978 and Ninth Revision for 1979-1984.

In this report, deaths from residential fires are defined as those with an underlying external cause of death coded according to the ICD as E890-E899 and with a location of injury coded as "0" (home) in the NCHS tapes on mortality data. Information in these tapes includes the decedent's age, sex, date of death, race (white, black, or other), and state of residence, and the state in which the death occurred.

Conflagrations (E890) are defined as uncontrolled fires in private dwellings; clothing ignitions (E893) are defined as fires caused by ignition of clothing. An additional 5%-9% of residential fires were due to miscellaneous or unspecified causes, identified in this report as "other fires." The latter category includes the following: other fires in unspecified buildings or structures (E891), fires not in buildings or structures (E892), ignition from highly inflammable materials (E894), controlled fires in private dwellings (E895), controlled fires in other unspecified buildings or structures (E896), controlled fires not in buildings or structures (E897), other unspecified fires and flames (E898), and other unspecified fires (E899).

Population estimates from the Bureau of the Census for 1978-1984 were used to compute rates (*4*). These data for the United States and for each of the NCHS regions (Northeast, Midwest, South, and West) were used to compute crude death rates (deaths from residential fires per 100,000 population). Crude death rates were used because they are very similar to the age-adjusted rates, which were computed by using the 1980 U.S. census as a standard. Regional rates that were determined by using as the numerator either the number of deaths that occurred in a region or the number of deaths of residents in a region were similar. Only regional rates compiled from deaths that occurred in the region were reported.

Results

From 1978 through 1984, an average of 4,897 persons died each year from residential fires (Table 1). The number of these deaths decreased from 5,401 in 1978 to 4,466 in 1984. A 21% reduction occurred in the overall annual residential fire-related death rate per 100,000 persons (from 2.4 in 1978 to 1.9 in 1984). Although more of these deaths occurred among males than females, the death rate per 100,000 males decreased 20%, from 3.0 in 1978 to 2.4 in 1984. The death rate per 100,000 females decreased 26%, from 1.9 in 1978 to 1.4 in 1984.

Blacks had the highest residential fire-related death rate. Whites and others had identical rates in 1978 and 1979. After 1980, however, the rate for whites was higher than that for others, except in 1984 when the rates for whites and others were similar. Between 1978 and 1984, the residential fire-related death rates decreased for all three groups: 19% for blacks, 25% for whites, and 25% for others. The South had the highest rates, and the West had the lowest (Table 1). In all regions, however, between 1978 and 1984 rates decreased 24% in the Northeast, 25% in the Midwest, 22% in the South, and 24% in the West.

TABLE 1. Number and rate of deaths from residential fires, by sex, race, and region, United States, 1978-1984

	1978		1979		1980		1981		1982		1983		1984	
	No.	Rate*	No.	Rate	No.	Rate	No.	Rate	No.	Rate	No.	Rate	No.	Rate
Sex														
Male	3,230	3.0	3,197	2.9	3,003	2.7	2,959	2.7	2,726	2.4	2,684	2.4	2,712	2.4
Female	2,171	1.9	2,102	1.8	2,080	1.8	1,997	1.7	1,836	1.5	1,828	1.5	1,754	1.4
Race														
White	3,785	2.0	3,645	1.9	3,550	1.8	3,382	1.7	3,155	1.6	3,028	1.5	2,997	1.5
Black	1,530	5.9	1,568	6.0	1,461	5.5	1,514	5.6	1,333	4.8	1,399	5.0	1,368	4.8
Other	86	2.0	86	1.9	72	1.4	60	1.1	74	1.2	85	1.3	101	1.5
Region														
Northeast	1,029	2.1	1,016	2.1	973	2.0	958	1.9	914	1.9	873	1.8	820	1.6
Midwest	1,418	2.4	1,445	2.5	1,271	2.2	1,170	2.0	1,117	1.9	1,041	1.8	1,089	1.8
South	2,303	3.2	2,188	2.9	2,239	3.0	2,283	3.0	1,936	2.5	2,092	2.7	2,008	2.5
West	651	1.6	650	1.5	600	1.4	545	1.2	595	1.3	506	1.1	549	1.2
Total deaths	5,401	2.4	5,299	2.4	5,083	2.2	4,956	2.2	4,562	2.0	4,512	1.9	4,466	1.9

*Deaths/100,000 population.

Persons ≥65 years old and children <5 years old had the highest death rates from residential fires (Figure 1). Rates declined up to ages 15-19, increased slightly at ages 20-24, leveled off at 25-39, and rose sharply after age 75. Blacks had higher death rates from residential fires in every age group than whites and others (Figure 2). Black children under age 5 had nearly a fourfold greater death rate than white children, and

FIGURE 1. Death rates from residential fires, by age group, United States, 1978-1984

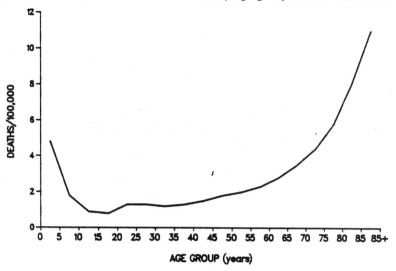

FIGURE 2. Death rates from residential fires, by age group and race, United States, 1978-1984

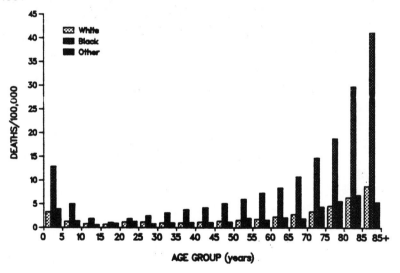

blacks over age 74 had death rates at least five times higher than those of whites and others in this age group. Persons listed as whites and others had similar death rates until age 84. After 84, the rate of whites exceeded that of others.

Deaths from residential fires are more common in the winter than in other seasons of the year (Figure 3). In this study, 40.1% of the deaths occurred during the winter, and only 14.2% occurred during the summer.

FIGURE 3. Distribution of deaths from residential fires, by season, United States, 1978-1984

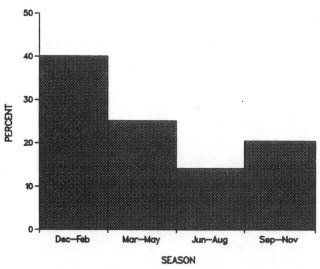

Most deaths from residential fires in the United States (86%-91%) are classified as conflagrations (Table 2). The remainder result from clothing ignition (3%-5%) and from other fires (5%-9%). For the U.S. population, the death rate from conflagrations decreased 19%—from 2.1/100,000 persons in 1978 to 1.7 in 1984. From 1979 through 1984, the death rate from clothing ignition remained stable at a rate of 0.1/100,000 persons, and the death rate from other fires decreased 43%. In 1984, the risk of dying from conflagrations was more than 21 times greater than the risk of dying in a residential fire from clothing ignition. By racial group, blacks had the highest death rates in every category of residential fire. Whites and others had similar rates, although in clothing ignition and other fires, the rates for other races should be interpreted with caution, since they were based on small numbers.

Discussion

The elderly, children <5 years old, and blacks of all ages are at high risk for death from residential fires. Most such deaths occur when a structure catches fire (conflagration), as opposed to burns from clothing ignition. Most deaths from residential fires occur in the winter, and the South is the region with the highest residential fire-related death rates.

The findings of this study have several limitations. First, the number of deaths reported here may be less than the true number of deaths from residential fires in the United States, because some fires in which the place of occurrence was undetermined (location coded as "9" on the death certificate) may have been residential. Second, the rates for blacks were not adjusted for the 1980 undercounted census report for that population (7.5% for black males and 2.1% for black females) (5). When the data were adjusted for this undercount, however, the results did not change appreciably. Third, the computation of regional rates was based on the number of

TABLE 2. Deaths and death rates from residential fires, by type of fire, year, and race, United States, 1978-1984

Year	White Deaths	White Rate*	Black Deaths	Black Rate	Other Deaths	Other Rate	Subtotal Deaths	Subtotal Rate
			Conflagrations (E890)					
1978	3,229	1.7	1,358	5.2	76	1.8	4,663	2.1
1979	3,192	1.6	1,407	5.3	79	1.7	4,678	2.1
1980	3,081	1.6	1,315	4.9	67	1.3	4,463	2.0
1981	3,030	1.5	1,393	5.1	55	1.0	4,478	2.0
1982	2,859	1.4	1,247	4.5	68	1.1	4,174	1.8
1983	2,643	1.3	1,254	4.5	76	1.2	3,973	1.7
1984	2,654	1.3	1,248	4.4	94	1.4	3,996	1.7
			Clothing ignition (E893)					
1978	203	0.1	58	0.2	4	0.1	265	0.1
1979	185	0.1	53	0.2	3	0.1	241	0.1
1980	195	0.1	60	0.2	2	0.0	257	0.1
1981	140	0.1	41	0.2	0	0.0	181	0.1
1982	116	0.1	30	0.1	2	0.0	148	0.1
1983	158	0.1	62	0.2	3	0.0	223	0.1
1984	143	0.1	43	0.2	0	0.0	186	0.1
			Other fires (E891, E892, E894-E899)					
1978	353	0.2	114	0.4	6	0.1	473	0.2
1979	268	0.1	108	0.4	4	0.1	380	0.2
1980	274	0.1	86	0.3	3	0.1	363	0.2
1981	212	0.1	80	0.3	5	0.1	297	0.1
1982	180	0.1	56	0.2	4	0.1	240	0.1
1983	227	0.1	83	0.3	6	0.1	316	0.1
1984	200	0.1	77	0.3	7	0.1	284	0.1

*Deaths/100,000 population.

deaths occurring in states that included some deaths of nonresidents. The findings were not appreciably affected, however, because such large populations (regional) were used as denominators. Therefore, the findings reported here provide a good estimate of death rates from residential fires.

An increased risk of dying in residential fires is associated with a number of human, environmental, and behavioral factors. The elderly and children are at increased risk, for example, partly because of the difficulty they may have in escaping from a house fire (6). The elderly are also less likely to own smoke detectors, as are blacks, the poor, and people who did not finish high school (7). Children are often at increased risk as a result of playing with matches (6). An increased risk for blacks may also be associated with poverty and with residence in older buildings (8), in rural areas, and in locations where the service of a fire department is delayed or unavailable (9).

More deaths from residential fires occur in winter than in other seasons of the year, possibly because of greater exposure to heating sources, improper installation and maintenance of wood- or coal-burning stoves, and the use of kerosene or space heaters (*9,10*). The use of kerosene and space heaters appears to be more common in the South (*9*). In addition, the winter season is shorter and milder there than in the Northeast or Midwest, and therefore space heaters may be more economical to use than central heating.

Behavioral risk factors also contribute to residential fires. These include cigarette smoking and alcohol use. Cigarettes are involved in half of the deaths caused by house fires (*9*), and cigarette-ignited fires typically occur at night when people fall asleep smoking in bed (*9*). Alcohol intoxication could hamper the chances of escape during a fire, and several investigations have indicated that 39%-43% of victims of residential fires who were tested for alcohol were legally intoxicated (blood alcohol concentration of ≥0.1 mg/dl) (*8,11*).

Various intervention strategies have been started to decrease the number of deaths from residential fires. The National Fire Protection Association collects and disseminates data on the estimated prevalence of fires, fire-related injuries, and fire-related property damage. The risk of dying from fires in homes with smoke detectors is half that in homes without detectors (*7*). The technology of smoke detectors was developed in the 1960s, but smoke detectors were not widely used until the 1980s, as suggested by national surveys on smoke detector ownership (5% in 1970 and 74% in 1985) (*7*). The increased ownership of smoke detectors may be the result of heightened public awareness of their safety value, a substantial decrease in smoke detector prices, and legislation requiring the installation of smoke detectors in homes (*7,12*).

Other intervention strategies have focused on improving the flame-retardant property of sleepwear (*13*), decreasing the number of cigarette smokers (*3*), and promoting self-extinguishing cigarettes and matches (*14*).

Since 1978, progress has been made in reducing deaths from residential fires. Overall rates have declined, although the elderly, children, blacks, and residents in the South remain at high risk.

The 1990 objective is limited as an indicator of the public health impact of residential fires. One overall crude death rate is used as an indicator of progress; therefore, the objective does not address the importance of specific high-risk populations. For example, the objective of 1.5 deaths/100,000 persons has been met or nearly met for females, whites, others, and residents of the Northeast, Midwest, and West. The objective is far from being met, however, for the elderly, children, and blacks. Unless particular attention is focused on effective interventions in these high-risk groups, the crude residential fire-related death rates may actually begin to increase. For example, the number of elderly people in the United States is expected to almost double by the year 2030 (from 11.6% in 1982 to 21.2 in 2030) (*15*).

The 1990 objective does not take nonfatal fire-related injuries into account. The Federal Emergency Management Agency, National Fire Protection Association, Consumer Product Safety Commission, and state, local, and nongovernmental agencies could jointly develop an objective that would reflect both mortality and morbidity. Such an objective would require the ability to collect reliable morbidity data that are currently unavailable.

To meet the 1990 objective concerning deaths from residential fires, health personnel need to increase their efforts to 1) examine high-risk groups, 2) develop a better surveillance system on the causes of fires, 3) implement effective interventions, and 4) evaluate intervention strategies. Further efforts toward attaining the 1990 objective should focus on increasing the use of smoke detectors, decreasing the number of persons who smoke, lowering the ignition potential of cigarettes, requiring that cigarettes and matches be self-extinguishing, and enforcing building codes related to fires.

References
1. National Safety Council. Accident facts 1985 edition. Chicago: National Safety Council, 1986.
2. Karter MJ Jr. Fire loss in the United States during 1984. Fire J 1985;Sept:14-25,67-75.
3. CDC. Mid-Course review report for the 1990 injury prevention objectives. Atlanta, Georgia: CDC, 1985.
4. US Department of Commerce, Bureau of the Census. Current population estimates and projections. Washington, DC: US Department of Commerce. (Series P-25, nos. 917, 1982; 957, 1984; 998, 1986; and 1,000, 1987.)
5. Savage IR. Who counts? Am Stat 1982;36:195-200.
6. Karter MJ Jr. Patterns of fire deaths among the elderly and children in the home. Fire J 1986;Mar:19-22.
7. Hall JR Jr. A decade of detectors: measuring the effect. Fire J 1985;Sept:37-43,78.
8. Mierley MC, Baker SP. Fatal house fires in an urban population. JAMA 1983;249:1466-8.
9. Baker SP, O 'Neill B, Karpf RS. The injury fact book. Lexington, Massachusetts: DC Heath, 1984:139-54.
10. Harwood B, Kluge P. Hazards associated with the use of wood- or coal-burning stoves or free-standing fireplaces. Washington, DC: US Consumer Product Safety Commission, 1985.
11. CDC. Deaths associated with fires, burns, and explosions—New Mexico, 1978-1983. MMWR 1985;34:623-5.
12. McLoughlin E, Marchone M, Hanger SL, German PS, Baker SP. Smoke detector legislation: its effect on owner-occupied homes. Am J Public Health 1985;75:858-62.
13. Robertson LS. Injuries: causes, control strategies, and public policy. Lexington, Massachusetts: DC Heath, 1983:153-4.
14. McGuire A. Cigarettes and fire deaths. NY State J Med 1983;83:1296-8.
15. US Department of Commerce, Bureau of the Census. Current population estimates and projections: projections of the population of the United States, by age, sex, and race: 1983 to 2080. Washington, DC: US Department of Commerce, 1984.

Regional Distribution of Deaths from Residential Fires — United States, 1978–1984

The week of October 4–10 marks the 65th anniversary of Fire Prevention Week, which was proclaimed by President Warren Harding in 1922 to commemorate the Great Chicago Fire of 1871. The objectives of Fire Prevention Week are to promote fire safety and prevent fire-related injuries, deaths, and property damage. Prevention activities focus on promoting safe storage of matches and flammable liquids, teaching children not to play with matches, and discouraging people from smoking in bed. Injury risk-reduction programs teach how to install and maintain smoke detectors, how to put out fires, and how to escape during a fire.

—MMWR Vol. 36/No. 39, October 9, 1987, pp. 645–9

Regional Distribution of Deaths
from Residential Fires — United States, 1978–1984

In 1984, 5,010 people in the United States lost their lives in fires; almost 90% of them died in residential fires (National Center for Health Statistics [NCHS], unpublished data). To assess the regional distribution of these deaths,* 1978-1984 mortality data collected by NCHS[†] were analyzed.

While an average of 4,897 persons died in residential fires each year during the period 1978-1984 (Table 1), residential fire death rates per 100,000 population decreased 21%, from 2.4 in 1978 to 1.9 in 1984 (CDC, unpublished data). The South had the largest average number of deaths per year (2,150) and the highest average death rate per 100,000 population (2.9). In contrast, the West had the lowest average number of deaths per year (585) and the lowest death rate per 100,000 population (1.4). Residential fire deaths and death rates for the Northeast and the Midwest were lower than those for the South, but higher than those for the West.

---

*Deaths from residential fires are those with the underlying cause of death coded as E890-E899 and place of occurrence coded as 'home,' based on the International Classification of Diseases, Supplementary Classification of External Cause of Injury, 8th Revision Adapted for 1978 and 9th Revision for 1979-1984.
[†]To compute sex- and age-specific death rates, the average annual number of deaths occurring during the period 1978-1984 in each of the four NCHS regions (Northeast, Midwest, South, and West) were used as a numerator, and the 1980 regional census total was used as the denominator.

TABLE 1. Average annual number of residential fire deaths and death rates* per 100,000 population, by sex and age of decedents and by type of fire — United States, 1978-1984

	South		Midwest		Northeast		West		Total[†]	
	No. Deaths	Rate	No. Deaths	Rate	No. Deaths	Rate	No. Deaths	Rate	No. Deaths	Rate
Sex										
Male	1,331	3.6	725	2.5	531	2.3	343	1.6	2,930	2.7
Female	819	2.1	497	1.6	410	1.6	242	1.1	1,967	1.7
Age										
<5 years	343	6.2	226	5.2	138	4.5	78	2.3	785	4.8
5-64 years	1,189	1.9	679	1.4	533	1.3	331	0.9	2,733	1.5
≥65 years	615	7.2	316	4.7	268	4.4	175	4.1	1,373	5.4
Type										
Conflagration	1,897	2.5	1,104	1.9	837	1.7	509	1.2	4,346	1.9
Clothing ignition	92	0.1	45	0.1	48	0.1	29	0.1	214	0.1
Other	161	0.2	72	0.1	56	0.1	47	0.1	336	0.1
Total deaths tabulated[†]	2,150	2.9	1,222	2.1	940	1.9	585	1.4	4,897	2.2

*(Total number of deaths, 1978-1984) ÷ 7
        1980 population
[†]Rows and columns may not equal total because of rounding.

Overall, males in the South had the most residential fire deaths and the highest death rate per 100,000. The male to female ratio of residential fire death rates varied by region from 1.4 to 1.7. However, death rates for females in the South were higher than for females in other regions and higher than for males in the West.

In all regions, residential fire death rates were much higher for children aged 0-4 years and the elderly (≥65 years) than for those aged 5-64 years; however, the rate differences were most pronounced in the South. Children had higher residential fire death rates than the elderly in the Midwest and the Northeast. However, in the South and West, residential fire death rates were lower for children than for the elderly.

For each region, deaths from conflagrations (uncontrolled fires) (E890) represented 87% to 90% of deaths from residential fires; those from clothing ignitions (E893) represented 4% to 5%; and those from other residential fires such as fires in unspecified buildings or structures (E891) and ignition from highly inflammable material (E894) represented 6% to 8%. For each type of residential fire death, the South had the highest number of deaths, and the West, the lowest. For conflagrations, the residential fire death rate was highest in the South (2.5) and lowest in the West (1.2); fire death rates were similar in the Northeast (1.7) and Midwest (1.9). For clothing ignition, the residential fire death rates were identical in all four regions (0.1). For all other residential fire deaths, the rate in the Northeast, Midwest, and West was 0.1; the rate in the South was 0.2.

Most residential fire deaths occurred in the winter (December-February), and the fewest occurred in the summer (June-August) (Figure 1). Within each region, the seasonal distribution of residential fire deaths varied markedly. In the winter, the number of deaths in every region was 1.5 to 3.3 times the number of deaths in the summer. For every season, the South had the highest number of deaths, and the West had the lowest.

FIGURE 1. Average annual residential fire deaths, by region and season — United States, 1978-1984

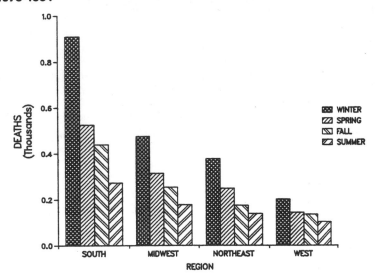

Reported by: Epidemiology Br, Div of Injury Epidemiology and Control, Center for Environmental Health and Injury Control, CDC.

Editorial note: The week of October 4-10 marks the 65th anniversary of Fire Prevention Week (FPW), which was first observed in 1922 after President Warren Harding proclaimed a national fire prevention day to commemorate the Great Chicago Fire of 1871 *(1)*. The Chicago fire destroyed over 17,000 buildings, killed 250 persons, and rendered 10,000 others homeless *(1)*.

Since residential fire deaths have accounted for most deaths from fires and flames in recent years, the U.S. Department of Health and Human Services identified residential fires as an important area for intervention and established an objective to reduce the death rate from the 2.4 deaths per 100,000 recorded in 1978 to 1.5 deaths per 100,000 by 1990 *(2)*. At the same time, the department established an objective to increase the number of functioning smoke detectors in residential homes from 30 million in 1979 to at least 110 million (75% of homes) by 1990 *(2)*. These objectives go hand-in-hand with the aim of FPW activities—to promote fire safety and prevent fire-related injuries, deaths, and property damage.

During FPW, individual fire departments across the nation conduct additional fire safety programs for targeted populations in their areas. These programs are of two general types: preventing fires from occurring and reducing the risk of injury in the event of fire. Prevention activities focus on promoting safe storage of matches and flammable liquids such as gasoline and kerosene, teaching children not to play with matches, and discouraging people from smoking in bed. Injury risk-reduction programs teach how to install and maintain smoke detectors, how to put out fires, and how to escape during a fire.

Smoke detectors are relatively inexpensive devices designed to warn people of a fire before it becomes unmanageable and noxious gases are released. Although the effectiveness of smoke detectors has not been thoroughly evaluated, one investigator estimated that the residential fire death rate in homes with a detector was half that in homes without one *(3)*. Possible explanations for continued residential fire deaths include the low prevalence of smoke detectors in the homes of high-risk groups and poor maintenance of smoke detectors after installation; personal characteristics such as alcohol consumption and smoking in bed; and conditions that hamper the chances of escape from a fire, such as hearing and/or visual impairment, the effect of medications, lack of mobility, or advanced age *(4-7)*. Additional risk factors for residential fires are poverty, poor housing, and decreased availability and slower response of fire department services *(7-9)*.

Reasons for the high rate of residential fire deaths in the South are not known because definitive studies on residential fires have not been conducted. There is, however, some evidence that, compared with other regions, the South has had a lower prevalence of smoke detectors *(10)*, a higher usage of portable heating equipment *(6)*, and a larger percentage of persons below the poverty level *(11)*. Together, these factors may contribute to the higher rate of residential fire deaths in the South.

The overall residential fire death rate in the West was lower than 1.5 deaths per 100,000 (the 1990 objective rate for residential fires), although children, the elderly, and males in this region had rates higher than 1.5. The overall death rates for all other regions were 27% to 93% higher than the 1990 objective, and some age-specific rates far exceeded the 1990 objective for lowering the residential fire death rate.

Most residential fire deaths occurred in the winter, followed by spring, fall, and summer. Since the risk of dying in a residential fire varies markedly by season, deaths from residential fires might be reduced if fire prevention and risk-reduction activities in each region target high-risk groups at appropriate times of the year. Residential fire death rates might be further reduced by increasing the prevalence of functioning smoke detectors in the homes of high-risk groups, by adopting safe house-heating practices, and by modifying commercial brands of cigarettes to reduce their potential to start fires on upholstered furniture or mattresses (12; National Bureau of Standards, unpublished data). The manufacture of self-extinguishing and otherwise less fire-prone cigarettes is technically feasible, according to a recent study conducted by the National Bureau of Standards (National Bureau of Standards, unpublished data).

The maintenance of functioning smoke detectors in high-risk homes will require innovative approaches. For example, to reduce fire death risks for the elderly, a public health nurse or a home health-care provider might be asked to check the condition of the smoke detector and complete a fire safety checklist as part of the medical evaluation. Further information is needed to assess the effectiveness of smoke detectors in homes of the elderly and to ascertain specific circumstances leading to residential fire deaths.

References

1. National Fire Protection Association. Develop and practice a home fire escape plan during NFPA's fire prevention week, October 4-10, 1987. Quincy, Massachusetts: National Fire Protection Association, 1987.
2. Public Health Service. Promoting health/preventing disease: objectives for the nation. Washington, DC: US Department of Health and Human Services, Public Health Service, 1980.
3. Hall JR Jr. A decade of detectors: measuring the effect. Fire Journal 1985;79:37-43, 78.
4. CDC. Prevalence of smoke detectors in private residences—DeKalb County, Georgia, 1985. MMWR 1986;35:445-8.
5. Karter MJ Jr. Patterns of fire deaths among the elderly and children in the home. Fire Journal 1986;Mar:19-22.
6. Baker SP, O'Neill B, Karpf RS. Burns and fire deaths. In: The injury fact book. Lexington, Massachusetts: Lexington Books, 1984:139-54.
7. Mierley MC, Baker SP. Fatal house fires in an urban population. JAMA 1983;249:1466-8.
8. Feck G, Baptiste MS, Tate CL Jr. An epidemiologic study of burn injuries and strategies for prevention. Atlanta: US Department of Health, Education, and Welfare, Public Health Service, 1978.
9. CDC. Deaths associated with fires, burns, and explosions—New Mexico, 1978-1983. MMWR 1985;34:623-5.
10. Hall JR Jr, Groeneman S. Two homes in three have detectors. Fire Service Today 1983;50:18-20.
11. Bureau of the Census. General social and economic characteristics. In: 1980 census of population. Washington, DC: US Department of Commerce, 1983; publication no. (PC)80-1-C1. (Vol 1).
12. Smith L. Consumer use of portable electric heaters—results of a national survey in April 1985. Washington, DC: US Consumer Product Safety Commission, 1986.

Deaths Associated with Fires, Burns, and Explosions — New Mexico, 1978–1983

Cigarette smoking, the use of natural or propane gas, and alcohol consumption all contributed to fire-related deaths in New Mexico. The New Mexico findings show an increased risk of fire-, burn-, and explosion-related deaths among American Indians.

—MMWR Vol. 34/No. 40, October 11, 1985, pp. 623–5

Deaths Associated with Fires, Burns, and Explosions — New Mexico, 1978–1983

The New Mexico Health and Environment Department (NMHED) examined fire-, burn-, and explosion-associated deaths occurring in the state during 1978-1983. Data were collected from death certificates recorded by the Vital Statistics Bureau of NMHED, death reports from the Office of the Medical Investigator (OMI), and fire-fatality reports from the New Mexico State Fire Marshal's Office. Included were all deaths caused unintentionally by fire and flames (E890-899), explosive material (E923), and hot substance or object, caustic or corrosive material, and steam (E924).* Also included were fire-associated deaths by suicide (E958.1) and assault (E968.1) and of undetermined intent (E988.1). Rates were calculated using 1980 census data for New Mexico. Ninety-four percent of persons whose deaths were coded as above were residents of New Mexico.

During 1978-1983, 204 deaths in New Mexico were identified as caused by fires, burns, or explosions. Of these deaths (identified from all three sources) 196 (97%) were identified in the OMI records; 195 (96%) were identified through death certificates listing cause of death; and 94 (46%) were found in the Fire Marshal records.

The average annual crude mortality rate was 2.6 per 100,000 persons (Table 2). The sex- and age-adjusted death rate for American Indians was twice that for white, non-Hispanics; the rate for persons of Hispanic origin was slightly higher than that for white, non-Hispanics.

TABLE 2. Adjusted annual mortality rates* from fires, burns, and explosions, by ethnicity — New Mexico, 1978-1983

Ethnicity	Deaths		Rate ratio
	No.	Rate	
White, non-Hispanic	107	2.3	1.0
Hispanic	73	2.9	1.2
American Indian	22	4.6	2.0
Other	2	—	
Total	**204**	**2.6**	

*Per 100,000 persons and adjusted to the age and sex distribution of 1980 New Mexico population.

Mortality rates varied by age, sex, and urban or rural location as defined by Standard Metropolitan Statistical Areas (SMSAs). The average annual age-adjusted death rate for males (4.0/100,000) was about three times that for females (1.4/100,000). Age-specific mortality rates were similar for males and females up to 14 years of age. Among persons older than 14 years, rates were higher for males than for females, with the highest rates for persons over age 75 years. The average annual death rate in the urbanized SMSAs (1.5/100,000) was 45% of that outside SMSAs (3.3/100,000).

Thirty (15%) of the New Mexico deaths occurred in the workplace, compared with 5%-6% nationally (1). Of the 30, 14 (47%) were caused by gas explosions (Table 3). Fires or explosions involving homes, mobile homes or other structures accounted for 119 deaths. Thirty-two (27%) of these deaths in homes or other structures occurred in mobile and trailer homes, which account for only 12% of year-round housing in New Mexico.

---

*Based on International Classification of Diseases, 9th Revision. Supplementary Classification of External Cause of Injury.

TABLE 3. Deaths from fires, burns, and explosions — New Mexico, 1978-1983

Situation	Deaths
Work-related	
Gas explosion	14
Oil refinery or well explosion or fire	4
Gas station fire	3
Mine explosion or fire	2
Fall into incinerator	2
Other	5
Subtotal	30
Nonwork-related	
House or other structure fire or explosion	119
Kitchen fire	3
Bedding fire	13
Clothing fire	22
Camping fire	1
Stationary auto fire or explosion	3
Scalding	9
Subtotal	170
Unknown	4
Total	204

Although not shown here, work-related deaths were equally distributed throughout the year; however, the frequency of nonwork-related deaths during winter months was twice that observed for the summer months.

Cigarette smoking, use of natural or propane gas, and alcohol consumption all contributed to fire-related deaths in New Mexico. Thirty-nine (19%) fire-related deaths were associated with cigarette smoking. Use of natural or propane gas was associated with 30 (15%) deaths. Blood alcohol concentrations (BAC) were measured at hospital admission or autopsy for 128 persons 10 years of age or older; 55 (43%) persons had BACs of 0.1 mg/dl or greater.

Reported by GA Conway, MD, formerly of the University of New Mexico School of Medicine, J Smialek, MD, M Starr, Office of the Medical Investigator, Albuquerque, T Langhorst, New Mexico State Fire Marshal's Office, T Ortiz, HF Hull, MD, State Epidemiologist, New Mexico Health and Environment Dept; Div of Injury Epidemiology and Control, Center for Environmental Health, CDC.

Editorial Note: The distribution of fire-, burn-, and explosion-related death rates by the age and sex of the victim in New Mexico is similar to that seen nationally (2,3). Rates are highest for males, preschool-aged children, and persons over 75 years of age. In addition, the seasonal distribution of deaths is consistent with national patterns. Home fires occur more frequently during winter months when heating is required and more time is spent indoors.

The New Mexico findings show an increased risk of fire-, burn-, and explosion-related deaths among American Indians, compared with that of other racial or ethnic groups. However, the risk for this group is similar to that for persons outside SMSAs. Ninety-five percent of fire-related deaths among American Indians in New Mexico occurred outside SMSAs. Reasons for this increased risk for fire fatality outside SMSAs may include decreased availability and response of fire department services, decreased likelihood of early discovery, less safe structures, and greater use of unsafe heating methods (2).

New Mexico has one of the lowest rates of mortality from house fires (2), possibly because of widespread use of materials other than wood, especially adobe, in home construction. In contrast, persons living in mobile homes in New Mexico have an increased risk of death from fires. Further study of mobile home dwellers would help identify risk factors and would, therefore, help target prevention programs. House-fire fatalities could be reduced by proper installation and maintenance of smoke detectors, regardless of structure type (4-6).

New Mexico has developed a model reporting system for injury surveillance based on collaboration between the state health department and organizations not often recognized as partners in public health. The OMI and Fire Marshal data provided important details surrounding the cause of death and identified 12 fire-related deaths not found by death certificates alone. The OMI in New Mexico is one of the first state medical examiner's offices to develop a computerized data system. As more such offices become computerized, all mortality surveillance, including injury surveillance, should improve.

References
1. National Safety Council. Accident facts, 1983. Chicago: National Safety Council, 1983.
2. Baker SP, O'Neill B, Karpf RS. The injury fact book. Lexington, Massachusetts: Lexington Books, 1984.
3. Feck G, Baptiste MS, Tate CL, Jr. An epidemiologic study of burn injuries and strategies for prevention. Atlanta, Georgia: U.S. Department of Health, Education, and Welfare, Public Health Service, Centers for Disease Control, January 1978.
4. Mierley MC, Baker SP. Fatal house fires in an urban population. JAMA 1983;249:1466-8.
5. McLoughlin E, Marchone M, Hanger SL, German PS, Baker SP. Smoke detector legislation: its effect on owner-occupied homes. Am J Public Health 1985;8:858-62.
6. Smith GS, Falk H, Coleman P. Unintentional injuries intervention strategies and their potential for reducing human losses. A position paper for the Carter Center "closing the gap" project. Atlanta, Georgia: Emory University, 1984.

Prevalence of Smoke Detectors in Private Residences — Dekalb County, Georgia, 1985

Results from this study suggest that, although many households have a smoke detector, adequate protection by these devices may be overestimated. Smoke detector protection should be a component of any community injury-control program, especially for older persons and other high-risk groups.

MMWR Vol. 35/No. 28, July 18, 1986, pp. 445–8

Prevalence of Smoke Detectors in Private Residences — Dekalb County, Georgia, 1985

To estimate the prevalence of smoke detectors in private residences in DeKalb County, Georgia (one of the several counties comprising greater Atlanta), and to ascertain factors associated with ownership, CDC conducted a county-wide random-digit-dialing telephone survey in July 1985 in cooperation with the DeKalb County Department of Public Safety, Fire Services, and the Georgia Department of Human Resources. Information requested included the following: whether a smoke detector was owned and installed; reasons for not owning a smoke detector; methods of testing the detector; residential and demographic characteristics of the respondent; and other data related to fire safety and prevention.

Interviews were conducted only if an adult household member (18 years of age or older) was available and if the household was a private residence. From a sampling frame including all phone numbers with DeKalb County prefixes, 2,477 numbers were randomly selected and called at least twice during one evening; 626 (25.3%) of these were eligible for inclusion. An additional 1,086 (43.8%) numbers were ineligible (due to nonworking numbers, business phones, or other reasons), and no one answered at 765 (30.9%) numbers. Of the 626 eligible residents contacted, 435 completed interviews.

Later, a random subsample of nonrespondent numbers was called up to 10 times to determine the characteristics of persons not reached in the original survey. Two-thirds of the numbers not contacted during the original survey were ineligible. Results of the callback survey were similar to those of the original survey for smoke detector ownership and other demographic characteristics (Table 1). Moreover, the original survey showed demographic characteristics similar to those based on U.S. Census Bureau data.

The prevalence of reported smoke detector ownership was 76.3%—comparable to the national average—although nearly 5% (15/332) of owned detectors were not reported to be installed (Table 1). Over half (57.9%) of the respondents reported owning fire extinguishers, and 65.7% also indicated having a fire escape plan for their dwelling.

TABLE 1. Characteristics of smoke detector survey sample and callback subsample — DeKalb County, Georgia, July 1985

Characteristic	Primary survey No.	Primary survey (%)	Callback subsample No.	Callback subsample (%)	Dekalb County 1980 U.S. Census (%)
Race of respondent: white	286	(65.7)	16	(72.7)	71.4
Education of respondent > high school	323	(74.3)	17	(77.3)	76.9
Child ≤ 5 yrs. old in dwelling	108	(24.8)	5	(22.7)	
Resident ≥ 65 yrs. old in dwelling	54	(12.4)	2	(9.1)	
Type of residence: "house"	301	(69.2)	14	(63.6)	
Dwelling > 10 yrs. old	297	(68.3)	17	(77.3)	68.7
Smoker in dwelling	191	(43.9)	9	(40.9)	
Smoke detector present in dwelling (1 or more)	332	(76.3)	18	(81.8)	
Installed smoke detector present in dwelling	317	(72.9)	18	(81.8)	
Fire extinguisher in dwelling	252	(57.9)	13	(59.1)	
Fire escape plan made	286	(65.7)	13	(72.7)	
Median age of respondent (yrs.)	28.0		33.5		29.1
Median no. residents per dwelling	3.0		2.5		2.8
Total	435	(100.0)	22		483,024

In dwellings under 10 years old, 89.9% had smoke detectors, compared with 71.8% in dwellings 10 years old or older (Table 2). Dwellings with residents over 65 years of age had an 18.3% lower prevalence of smoke detector ownership (64.1%) than those not so characterized (78.5%).

TABLE 2. Factors significantly associated with smoke detector ownership — Dekalb County, Georgia, July 1985

Characteristic	Response	Prevalence*	(%)	Prevalance ratio	p value
Age of dwelling	< 10 yrs. old	98/109	(89.9%)	1.25	< 0.001
	≥ 10 yrs. old	212/295	(71.8%)		
Resident ≥ 65	yes	34/53	(64.1%)	0.82	< 0.033
yrs. old in dwelling	no	295/376	(78.5%)		
Fire extinguisher	yes	213/251	(84.9%)	1.31	< 0.001
in dwelling	no	116/179	(64.8%)		
Respondent believes	yes	321/412	(77.9%)	2.34	< 0.006
smoke detectors	no	3/9	(33.3%)		
save lives					

*Number of respondents with smoke detectors divided by total number of respondents characterized by each value (excludes "don't know" category).

Nearly 85% of residents owning fire extinguishers also owned smoke detectors, while 64.8% of residents without fire extinguishers owned smoke detectors. Households in which the respondent believed that smoke detectors save lives were over twice as likely than other households to own smoke detectors (77.9 compared with 33.3%).

Characteristics not significantly associated with smoke detector ownership included sex and race of respondent, education level of head of household, ownership of dwelling, presence of a child 5 years of age or younger, a smoker in residence, type of dwelling, and a fire escape plan.

Although 121 (37.9%) of 319 of the sample of smoke detector owners tested their detectors at least once a month, 19.7% said they had never tested the devices. The remaining 47.3% of owners tested theirs less than once a month. The most frequently used manner of testing (40.3%) was by activating a button on the detector. Another 27.3% of respondents tested the detector by smoke challenge; 16.9% used both methods. The remaining respondents who tested used other methods. In a nonrandom home inspection follow-up of 10.6% of the original phone survey responders, nearly 30% of the owners had nonfunctioning smoke detectors, although they reported having an installed detector in their home.

The most common reasons for not owning smoke detectors were: "keep forgetting/putting off" (51.5%); "no interest/never thought about it" (37.8%); "not my responsibility" (24.0%); and "cost" (15.8%).

Reported by GN Bohan, MD, DeKalb County District No. 3, Unit No. 5, Capt CL Varnadoe, DeKalb County Dept of Public Safety, Fire Svcs, RK Sikes, DVM, State Epidemiologist, Georgia Dept of Human Resources; JR Hall, Jr, PhD, Fire Analysis Div, National Fire Protection Association, Quincy, Massachusetts; Div of Injury Epidemiology and Control, Center for Environmental Health, Div of Nutrition, Center for Health Promotion and Education, Div of Surveillance and Epidemiologic Studies, Epidemiology Program Office, Epidemic Intelligence Service Class of 1985, CDC.

Editorial Note: Every year in the United States, more than 4,000 deaths and 20,000 injuries result from residential fires (*1*). Many of these deaths and injuries occur at night while the victims are asleep and result from smoke and gas inhalation rather than flames. A study of deaths due to house fires in 1980, for example, showed that 66% were attributable to carbon monoxide or unspecified fumes (*2*).

Smoke detectors are a reliable method of awakening people before air becomes unbreathable from the buildup of smoke, carbon monoxide, and other toxic gases (*3*). Thus, these devices should allow more people to escape uninjured from house fires. The U.S. Fire Administration's National Fire Incident Reporting System (NFIRS) has estimated that a person who has a home fire and does not have a detector is twice as likely to die in that fire as a person protected by detectors (*4*).

The prevalence of smoke detectors in the United States. has been steadily increasing since the early 1970s, when only about 5% of households had them (*4*). By 1985, an estimated 75% of households had at least one smoke detector. Similarly, during 1978-1984, deaths from house fires dropped more than 30%, from 6,015 to 4,075. This decline is attributed in part to recent home fire safety efforts, including the passage of numerous state laws requiring the installation of smoke detectors (*1*). However, significant differences in the level of ownership among geographic regions exist. States in the South, for example, have the lowest prevalence of smoke detector ownership, although they have the highest fire fatality rates (*4*).

Results from this study suggest that, although many households have a smoke detector, adequate protection by these devices may be overestimated. Nonoptimal protection can be inferred from several findings: (1) 15 (4.5%) of the 332 households with smoke detectors did not have them installed; (2) 19.7% of owners never tested their smoke detectors, and on inspection, nearly 30% of the installed detectors were nonfunctioning; and (3) households with at least one smoke detector may not have all the smoke detectors needed or may have them improperly placed.

Finally, death rates from house fires are highest among older persons. This study also suggests that, even if the overall level of smoke detector prevalence in a community is high, this high-risk subgroup has a lower rate of ownership than other groups in DeKalb County. Results from a recent study suggest that the elderly, the poor, people who did not finish high school, and other groups at high risk of dying in a fire have been less likely to obtain detectors (*4*). Nonwhite households also have a lower prevalence of detectors than white households (*5*). (The differences in percentage of detector ownership by race and by education level of the head of the household in the national study were not found in the DeKalb County study; this may have been due to the size of the sample compared with the national surveys.)

Smoke detector protection should be a component of any community injury-control program, especially for older persons and other high-risk groups. It is inadequate to limit such a program solely to handing out smoke detectors. Proper installation and frequent testing are necessary to ensure adequate protection. Also, an important component is educating individuals on how best to use the extra escape time provided by their detectors. This includes not only creating an escape plan to be used in a fire, but also rehearsing that plan (*4*).

References
1. Hall JR. A decade of detectors: measuring the effect. Fire Journal 1985 (September):37-78.
2. Karter MJ. Fire loss in the United States during 1984. Fire Journal 1985 (September):14-76.
3. Baker SP, O'Neill B, Karpf R. Burns and fire deaths. The injury fact book. Lexington, Massachusetts: Lexington Books, 1984:139-54..
4. U.S. Consumer Product Safety Commission. What you should know about smoke detectors. Washington, D.C.: U.S. Consumer Product Safety Commission, 1983.
5. Hall JR, Jr, Groeneman S. Two homes in three have detectors. Fire Service Today 1983 (February): 18-20.

Hospitalizations Due to Tap Water Scalds, 1978–1985

More than 2,600 people sustain tap water scald burns each year. The majority of these injuries are directly related to inappropriate or inadvertent exposure to tap water heated to an excessive temperature. Primary prevention measures are based on three strategies: 1) increase public knowledge about the danger of hot tap water, 2) measure water temperature at the tap, and 3) reduce water temperature to 120° F by lowering the setting of water heater thermostats.

—MMWR Vol. 37/No. SS-1, February 1988, pp. 35–38

Hospitalizations Due to Tap Water Scalds, 1978–1985

Philip L. Graitcer, D.M.D., M.P.H.
Joseph E. Sniezek, M.D., M.P.H.
Progam Development and Implementation Branch
Division of Injury Epidemiology and Control
Center for Environmental Health and Injury Control

Introduction

Each year, approximately 112,000 people with scald burns are treated in hospital emergency rooms; approximately 6% of them are hospitalized. More than 2,600 of these burns are caused by hot tap water. Generally, tap water burns are more severe and extensive than other scald burns, and about 25% of the patients with these burns require hospitalization (*1*). Household water heaters that have been set at temperatures above 120° F (48.9° C) cause many of these tap water burns (*2*).

Young children, the elderly, and the physically impaired account for approximately 85% of hot tap water burns (*3*). Scalds often occur when infants or other young children are put into bathtubs in which the water is excessively hot, and they are unable to remove themselves. Similarly, the elderly and the handicapped are often unable to remove themselves from excessively hot water. Elderly persons have an increased risk for serious injury from burns because their skin has a reduced sensitivity to temperature.

In the light of these findings, and to reduce the incidence of what is considered an easily preventable problem, the U.S. Department of Health and Human Services set the following objective in 1979: "By 1990, the number of tap water scald injuries requiring hospital care should be reduced to no more than 2,000 per year." In 1978, the estimated number was 4,000 per year.

Methods

Accurate nationwide data sources are not available for determining the number of hospitalizations due to tap water scalds. Until 1984, the U.S. Consumer Product Safety Commission's National Electronic Injury Surveillance System (NEISS) provided estimates of the number of emergency room visits for hot water scalds. However, because of changes in the NEISS sampling design and in product injury coding in 1984, NEISS is no longer an appropriate source of data for such scalds. As a result, although the number of hot water scalds reported through NEISS has declined dramatically, this decline is artifactual. Tap water scalds are a portion of all hot water scalds.

The 1985 Health Interview Survey conducted by the National Center for Health Statistics (NCHS) provides nationwide population-based data about awareness of preventive measures for tap water scalds. Local and regional studies of scald injuries provide additional epidemiologic data. Although these studies have described risk groups and environmental factors affecting tap water scalds, the study results cannot be reliably extrapolated to derive national estimates.

Results

Based on NEISS data, the estimated number of hospital emergency room visits for scald injuries in the United States decreased slightly from 1978 to 1984. Each year, hot water scalds accounted for about half of these emergency visits (Table 1).

TABLE 1. Hospital emergency room visits and hospitalizations for scald injuries, by year, United States, selected years

	Year	All scald injuries	Hot water scalds
Emergency room visits	1983	133,516	69,863
	1984	129,238	65,843
Hospitalizations	1978	*	4,000
	1983	7,079	4,738
	1984	6,403	4,270

*Not available

Source: Consumer Product Safety Commission, National Electronic Injury Surveillance System (NEISS).

In the NCHS Health Interview Survey, 36.2% of the persons surveyed reported that they knew the temperature of the hot water in their homes (4). When asked how they estimated this temperature, 62.9% said that they used the setting on the water heater, 25.7% "guessed" the temperature, and 4.0% tested it with a thermometer. In households with children, compared with households without children, respondents had slightly more knowledge about tap water scalds and how to prevent them.

Local studies of tap water scalds help to identify risk factors. In Dane County, Wisconsin, risk factors were identified for 88% of the patients hospitalized for tap water scalds. Of the hospitalized patients, >50% were children <5 years of age, 9% were >65 years, and 30% were physically or mentally disabled (1). Almost all of these injuries could have been prevented by lowering the temperature of the household water heater to 120° F.

Discussion

The lack of a nationwide source of morbidity data hampers the accurate tracking of the 1990 objective concerning tap water scalds. Because of significant changes in NEISS, obtaining future usable data through this system is unlikely. NCHS Health Interview Survey data show that families reportedly know that high water temperatures can cause severe burns; however, these are self-reported data, and the interviewers do not actually measure water temperatures. Few households reported actually measuring their hot water temperature (4).

Local and regional studies of scald injuries have provided an epidemiologic basis for characterizing these injuries. Local data can help public health personnel determine target groups, identify risk factors, and find possible interventions. Local and regional studies have shown that residential water heaters with temperature settings above 120° F are the principal cause of tap water scalds.

A New Zealand retrospective study identified the child's environment as being the most important risk factor for scald injuries, although supervision of children did not appear to be a risk factor for hot water injuries (5). Child abuse has been implicated as another cause of tap water scalds; however, no published studies have quantified this risk.

The majority of tap water scald injuries are directly related to inappropriate or inadvertent exposure to tap water heated to an excessive temperature. Primary preventive measures are based on three strategies: 1) increase public knowledge about the danger of hot tap water, 2) measure water temperature at the tap, and 3) reduce water temperature to 120° F by lowering the setting of water heater thermostats.

Several community-sponsored programs are based on these strategies. In the Liberty City area of Miami, Florida, community injury control workers visited households, measured tap water temperature, and, if necessary, reduced the water temperature (Ros A. and Devito C., personal communication). These workers also discussed the dangers of hot tap water with parents of young children and with the elderly. In southern Wisconsin, the Wisconsin Electric Power Company distributed (with each electric bill) a brochure that described the danger and cost of excessively hot water. Each subscriber was offered a free liquid-crystal thermometer to use for testing hot water temperature at the tap. Of the approximately 750,000 subscribers, 140,211 requested thermometers. During the same period, a public information campaign was conducted, and messages were transmitted by radio and television to inform the public about hot tap water burns. A follow-up telephone evaluation indicated that after the campaign, nearly 90% of the general population was aware that tap water could cause severe burns in just seconds (6). Although changes in the number of tap water scalds were not measured in these campaigns, the informational activities demonstrably increased the public's awareness that excessively hot tap water can cause severe injuries.

Other approaches to reducing the number of tap water scalds also focus on reducing tap water temperature. Local ordinances have been proposed in some areas to establish a maximum tap water temperature in public buildings, but the effectiveness of such ordinances may be marginal since most scalds occur in the home. Some pediatricians have recommended that manufacturers preset thermostats on water heaters before shipping them from the factory. These manufacturers could also provide warning labels about the risk of higher temperatures (2). Wisconsin and Washington have legislation requiring manufacturers of home water heaters to set the thermostats at a safe level (Weiss H. and Rivara F., personal communication).

Although tap water scalds produce serious injuries in young children, the elderly, and the handicapped or physically impaired, the relatively small number of tap water scalds per year makes these injuries less of a public health problem than many other household injuries. For example, from 1978-1983, about 4,000-5,000 persons were hospitalized each year for hot water scalds, whereas 5,000 persons died each year in residential fires.

Since a distinct causative agent (excessively hot tap water) and several intervention strategies exist, reducing the number of tap water scalds is clearly an attainable objective. The lack of a nationwide data source, however, prevents the measurement of a reduction. Because the number of hospitalizations due to hot water scalds is small, data from the National Hospital Discharge Survey are not adequate for tracking this objective (7). Alternative data sources for national surveillance of tap water scalds need to be explored. Consideration may be given to reevaluating the tracking of this 1990 objective. Efforts to prevent tap water scalds should not be diminished, however, since the intervention is simple, cost beneficial, effective, and easily implemented.

References
1. Katcher ML. Scald burns from hot tap water. JAMA 1981;246:1219-22.
2. Feldman KW, Schaller RT, Feldman JA, McMillon M. Tap water scald burns in children. Pediatrics 1978;62:1-7.
3. Katcher ML, Delventhal SJ. Burn injuries in Wisconsin: epidemiology and prevention. Wis Med J 1982;81:25-8.
4. Hoffman RE. Tracking 1990 objectives for injury prevention with 1985 NHIS findings. Public Health Rep 1986;101:581-6.
5. Langley J, Dodge J, Silva PA. Scalds to preschool children. NZ Med J 1981;93:84-7.
6. Katcher ML. Prevention of tap water scald burns: evaluation of a multi-media control program. Presented at the 24th annual meeting of the Ambulatory Pediatric Association, San Francisco, California, May 1984.
7. National Center for Health Statistics, Graves EJ. Utilization of short stay hospitals, United States—1985. Hyattsville, Maryland: National Center for Health Statistics, May 1987; DHHS publication no. (PHS)87-1752. (Vital and health statistics; series 13, no. 91).

Sports and Leisure Activities

Alcohol Use and Aquatic Activities — United States, 1991

Because alcohol affects balance, movement, and vision, its use represents a risk for injury death for boat operators and passengers, who can fall overboard while intoxicated. Possible strategies to prevent alcohol-related aquatic injuries include eliminating advertisements that encourage the use of alcohol during boating activities and restricting the sale of alcoholic beverages at aquatic facilities.

—MMWR Vol. 42/No. 35, September 10, 1993, pp. 675, 681–3

Alcohol Use and Aquatic Activities — United States, 1991

Drowning, a leading cause of death from unintentional injury in the United States, accounted for approximately 4600 fatalities in 1991 (*1,2*). Although 25%–50% of adolescents and adults who drowned had consumed alcohol near the time of death (*3*), information regarding drinking behaviors during aquatic activities is limited. To assist in refining strategies for prevention of alcohol-related injury in aquatic settings, during July 15–September 30, 1991, the Boston University School of Public Health surveyed a national sample of adolescents and adults regarding their participation in aquatic activities and associated alcohol use. This report summarizes these findings.

The two-stage Waksberg random-digit–dialing telephone procedure was used to obtain a probability sample of working residential telephone numbers in the continental United States (*4,5*). One randomly designated respondent aged ≥16 years was selected from each household. Of 3042 households contacted, 2706 persons (89%; 1255 [46%] men; 1451 [54%] women) reported participation in at least one activity on or near the water during the year preceding the interview and participated in the survey. Respondents were aged 16–94 years (mean: 42 years; median: 39 years). The standard error does not exceed ±2% for any given point estimate in this study. The most frequently reported aquatic activities were swimming (75%) and boating (72%).

Respondents were asked about alcohol use during participation in aquatic activities during the year preceding the interview. Of the 2706 respondents, 1889 (70%; 926 [74%] males; 963 [66%] females) reported alcohol use, and 817 (30%) abstained. Of the 1889 alcohol users, 1156 (61%; 656 [52%] males; 500 [34%] females) had consumed alcohol on at least one occasion while participating in an aquatic activity. The likelihood of having consumed alcohol varied by type of aquatic activity: of 2031 swimmers and 1943 boaters, 487 (24%) and 630 (32%), respectively, reported having used alcohol during those activities during the preceding year.

Respondents who participated in an aquatic activity during the 30 days preceding the interview (n=1877) were asked about associated alcohol use during their last day on or near the water. Of the 1877 respondents, 522 (28%) reported consuming alcohol during their last day of water recreation: 366 (70%) drank beer; 112 (21%), wine; 82 (16%), liquor; and 16 (3%), some other alcoholic beverage. Men who drank reported consuming more (mean: 4.5 alcoholic beverages) than did women (mean: 2.9 alcoholic beverages) on this occasion (p<0.0001) (Figure 1).

Of respondents who reported ever consuming alcohol during their lifetimes during aquatic activities (n=1183), 108 (9%) reported that they always or often drank on these occasions, 426 (36%) that they sometimes drank; and 649 (55%) that they rarely drank during aquatic activities. Two percent reported that alcohol consumption substantially increased their enjoyment of being on or near the water; 18%, "somewhat;" 23%, "a little;" and 56% reported that alcohol did not increase their enjoyment of being on or near the water.

Of the 3042 respondents, 2213 (73%) recalled at least one exposure to information (i.e., hearing or reading) about the risks of drinking during aquatic activities. A total of 2889 (95%) respondents strongly or somewhat favored laws for their own states that prohibit operation of recreational and commercial water vessels while intoxicated. In comparison, 34% and 42% of all respondents and respondents who had participated in boating, respectively, had knowledge of the 1984 legislation amending Title 46, United States Code, Chapter 23 (Operation of Vessels Generally), to include specific prohibitions regarding the operation of a vessel while intoxicated.

FIGURE 1. Mean number of alcoholic beverages consumed during the last day on or near the water by persons who participated in an aquatic activity during the 30 days preceding the interview, by sex and age group — United States, 1991*

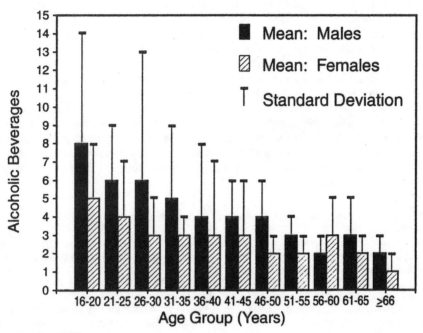

*Sample size=1877.

Reported by: J Howland, PhD, R Hingson, ScD, T Heeren, PhD, S Bak, MPH, Boston Univ School of Public Health; T Mangione, PhD, JSI Research and Training Institute. Epidemiology Br, National Center for Injury Prevention and Control, CDC.

Editorial Note: The determination that alcohol use is a risk factor for water-recreation–related fatalities is well documented (*6,7*). Alcohol use is a risk factor for injury and death in aquatic settings for a variety of reasons. For example, alcohol can reduce body temperature and, through its effect on the central nervous system, can impair swimming ability (*3*). In the national study described in this report, one third of boaters reported consuming alcohol while boating—a finding similar to one reported in the 1989 American Red Cross National Boating Survey (*8*), in which 29% of all boaters reported consuming alcohol during a typical boat outing. Because alcohol affects balance, movement, and vision, its use represents a risk for injury and death for boat operators and passengers, who can fall overboard while intoxicated (*3,9*).

The male-to-female ratio of drowning rates in the United States is approximately 14:1 for drownings associated with boating and 5:1 for other drownings (*1*). Alcohol use contributes largely to the sex differential in annual drowning rates. In the findings in this report, half of men and one third of women reported alcohol use during aquatic activities, and men reported consuming significantly more alcohol than did women, suggesting that sex differences in drowning may be related to differences in alcohol use and consumption.

More than half of all respondents reported that drinking did not increase their enjoyment of aquatic activities, and nearly all favored legislation that prohibits alcohol use in aquatic settings. These findings should assist in planning or refining strategies for prevention of alcohol-related injury in aquatic settings. In addition, only one third of respondents were aware of federal laws prohibiting the operation of a recreational boat while under the influence of alcohol, suggesting that alcohol advertisements involving aquatic settings may contribute to misconceptions about the safety and legality of combining alcohol use with swimming and boating (1).

Possible strategies for the prevention of alcohol-related aquatic injuries include 1) public service announcements by federal and state government agencies and community-based organizations warning about the dangers of combining alcohol use with water recreation: such messages should be tailored to swimming and boating; 2) elimination of advertisements that encourage the use of alcohol during boating activities; 3) restriction of sale of alcoholic beverages at aquatic facilities; and 4) passage and enforcement of federal and state legislation restricting water-recreation activities during alcohol consumption.

References
1. Baker SP, O'Neill B, Ginsburg MJ, Li G. The injury fact book. 2nd ed. New York: Oxford University Press, 1992.
2. National Safety Council. Accident facts. 1992 ed. Itasca, Illinois: National Safety Council, 1992.
3. Howland J, Hingson R. Alcohol as a risk factor for drowning: a review of the literature (1950–1985). Accid Anal Prev 1988;20:19–25.
4. CDC. Alcohol use and aquatic activities—Massachusetts, 1988. MMWR 1990;39:332–4.
5. Waksberg J. Sampling methods for random digit dialing. J Am Stat Assoc 1978;73:40–6.
6. Howland J, Mangione T, Hingson R, Levenson S, Winter M. A pilot survey of aquatic activities and related consumption of alcohol, with implications for drowning. Public Health Rep 1990;105:415–9.
7. CDC. Recreational boating fatalities—Ohio, 1983–1986. MMWR 1987;36:321–4.
8. American Red Cross. American Red Cross National Boating Survey: a study of recreational boats, boaters, and accidents in the United States. Washington, DC: American Red Cross, 1991.
9. Howland J, Smith GS, Mangione T, Hingson R, DeJong W, Bell N. Missing the boat on drinking and boating. JAMA 1993;270:91–2.

Alcohol Use and Aquatic Activities — Massachusetts, 1988

The prevalence of alcohol use during aquatic activities was high in this study—a finding that suggests the need to strengthen education about the risks of alcohol use and drowning in all aquatic environments.

—MMWR Vol. 39/No. 20, May 25, 1990, pp. 332–4

Alcohol Use and Aquatic Activities — Massachusetts, 1988

More than 8000 drowning fatalities occur in the United States each year, making drowning the third most common cause of death from unintentional injury in the United States (1,2). Although 25%–50% of adult and adolescent drowning victims had consumed alcohol near the time of death (3), information regarding drinking behaviors during aquatic activities is limited. In September 1988, the Boston University School of Public Health surveyed Massachusetts adults aged ≥20 years to determine in what settings and how often they consumed alcoholic beverages on or near the water during their most recent aquatic activity in August 1988.

A statewide probability sample was conducted through a random-digit-dialing procedure (4). Of 306 adults called, 294 (96%) participated in the survey. A total of 221 (75%; 107 [79%] men, 114 [72%] women) respondents reported a mean of 13 days of aquatic activities during August 1988. The most frequently reported aquatic activity was swimming (169 [76%]), followed by boating (55 [25%]), and fishing from shore (31 [14%]). The most frequently reported site of activity was the ocean (120 [54%]), followed by lakes or ponds (57 [26%]), pools (38 [17%]), rivers (five [2%]), and other settings (1 [<1%]).

Of persons reporting aquatic activities, 38 (36%) men and 13 (11%) women reported that they had consumed alcohol on the last occasion. Among alcohol users, 15 (29%) reported having consumed ≥4 drinks from 2 hours before until completion of the activity. Men who drank reported consuming more (mean: 3.5 drinks) than women (mean: 2.4 drinks) in an aquatic setting. The proportion of drinking did not vary substantially by location or activity. Respondents aged ≥50 years were less likely than younger respondents to report drinking on the last occasion on or near the water (Table 1).

Reported by: J Howland, PhD, R Hingson, ScD, S Levenson, MPH, M Winter, Boston Univ School of Public Health; T Mangione, PhD, Center for Survey Research, Univ of Massachusetts at Boston. Unintentional Injuries Section, Epidemiology Br, Div of Injury Control, Center for Environmental Health and Injury Control, CDC.

Editorial Note: The relationship between alcohol use and water recreation fatalities has been documented in a variety of settings (1,5,6). For example, the National Transportation Safety Board estimated that alcohol use was associated with 32%–64% of recreational boating deaths in 1983 (7,8). In a North Carolina study of drownings from 1980 through 1984, 399 (46%) of 869 drowning victims ≥15 years of age tested positive for blood alcohol, and 286 (33%) had blood alcohol concentrations (BACs) of >0.1 g/dL (1).

The ratio of male-to-female drowning rates in the United States is approximately 12:1 for drownings associated with boating and approximately 5:1 for other drownings (9); the gender difference in drowning rates does not change with age (10–12). The Massachusetts data suggest that differences by sex in aquatic-activity–related morbidity and mortality may be associated with differences in behaviors (e.g., use of alcohol, use of personal flotation devices, and participation in different types of water activities [13]) rather than exposure to aquatic environments. Men are more likely than women to drink alcohol on or near the water.

In the United States, more than 50 million persons engage in various recreational (noncommercial) boating activities on at least 8 days per year (5,6), and 90% of all deaths from recreational boating result from drowning. The prevalence of alcohol use during aquatic activities in Massachusetts was high when compared with the estimated prevalence of alcohol exposure among weekend nighttime drivers, who have the highest overall estimate known among U.S. drivers (8.3% of a 1983 U.S. driver sample had BACs of ≥0.1 g/dL) (2). This information suggests the need to 1) strengthen education about the risks of drowning in all aquatic environments and 2) clarify the relationship between alcohol use, drowning, and other water recreation injuries.

TABLE 1. Number and percentage of 221 surveyed adults who drank alcohol during their most recent aquatic activity, by sex, age group, location, and activity — Massachusetts, August 1988

Characteristic	No. reporting aquatic activity	Consuming alcohol		
		No.	(%)	95% CI*
Sex				
Male	107	38	(36)	27–45
Female	114	13	(11)	5–17
Age group (yrs)				
20–29	72	20	(28)	18–38
30–39	61	14	(23)	12–32
40–49	45	13	(29)	17–43
50–59	21	1	(5)	0–18
60–64	8	0		
≥65	12	2	(17)	0–38
Location				
River	5	2	(40)	25–47
Lake/pond	57	17	(30)	17–41
Pool	38	8	(21)	15–29
Ocean	120	24	(20)	13–27
Activity				
Power boating	55	17	(31)	19–43
Sailing	20	5	(25)	8–46
Swimming	169	44	(26)	19–33
Fishing from shore	31	7	(23)	8–38
Sun bathing	162	38	(23)	17–29
Fishing from boat	25	5	(20)	6–38
Total	221	51	(23)	

*Confidence interval.

References
1. Patetta MJ, Biddinger PW. Characteristics of drowning deaths in North Carolina. Public Health Rep 1988;103:406–11.
2. Brooks JG. Near drowning. Pediatr Rev 1988;10:5–10.
3. Howland J, Hingson R. Alcohol as a risk factor for drowning: a review of the literature (1950–1985). Accid Anal Prev 1988;20:19–25.
4. Waksberg J. Sampling methods for random digit dialing. J Am Stat Assoc 1978;73:40–6.
5. CDC. Recreational boating fatalities—Ohio, 1983–1986. MMWR 1987;36:321–4.
6. Smith GS, Kraus JF. Alcohol and residential, recreational and occupational injuries: a review of the epidemiologic evidence. Annu Rev Public Health 1988;9:99–121.
7. Wright SJ. SOS: alcohol, drugs and boating. Alcohol Health and Research World 1985; 9:28–33.
8. National Transportation Safety Board. Safety study: recreational boating safety and alcohol. Washington, DC: National Transportation Safety Board, 1983; publication no. NTSB no. SS-83-02.
9. Baker SP, O'Neill B, Karpf RS. The injury fact book. Lexington, Massachusetts: DC Heath and Co, 1984:156.
10. O'Carroll PW, Alkon E, Weiss B. Drowning mortality in Los Angeles County, 1976 to 1984. JAMA 1988;260:380–3.
11. Quan L, Gore EJ, Wentz K, Allen J, Novack AH. Ten-year study of pediatric drownings and near-drownings in King County, Washington: lessons in injury prevention. Pediatrics 1989;83:1035–40.
12. Wintemute GJ, Kraus JF, Teret SP, Wright MA. The epidemiology of drownings in adulthood: implications for prevention. Am J Prev Med 1988;4:343–8.
13. Gulaid JA, Sattin RW. Drownings in the United States, 1978–1984. In: Public health surveillance of 1990 injury control objectives for the nation. MMWR 1988;37(no. SS-1): 27–33.

Child Drownings and Near Drownings Associated with Swimming Pools — Maricopa County, Arizona, 1988 and 1989

From January 1988 through December 1989, fire departments in Maricopa County recorded 243 calls for drownings and near drownings involving children 4 years of age and younger. Measures to reduce childhood drownings and near drownings at swimming pools have included mandatory fencing and barriers around swimming pools.

—MMWR Vol. 39/No. 26, July 6, 1990, pp. 441–2

Child Drownings and Near Drownings Associated with Swimming Pools — Maricopa County, Arizona, 1988 and 1989

In Arizona, drowning* is a leading cause of fatal injuries among children ≤4 years of age (*1*). From 1981 to 1988, the annual rate of death from drowning for children in Arizona ranged from 9 to 15 per 100,000 children ≤4 years of age; from 1985 to 1987, the average annual rate for the United States was 4 per 100,000 children in this age group.

In April 1988, to help characterize the problem and to identify opportunities for intervention, the Arizona Department of Health Services requested that fire departments in Maricopa County (the Phoenix Standard Metropolitan Statistical Area; population, approximately 2 million) use a standard form to report drowning and near-drowning† incidents. In Maricopa County, fire departments are the first responders to 911 emergency telephone calls. From January 1988 through December 1989, fire departments recorded 243 calls for drownings and near drownings involving children ≤4 years of age. Of these, 206 (85%) occurred in swimming pools (Maricopa County has an estimated 125,000 public and private swimming pools); 23 (9%), in bathtubs; and 14 (6%), in other bodies of water (e.g., buckets, toilets, and ponds). Of the 206 swimming pool incidents, 111 (54%) occurred from May through August. Detailed report forms were available for 137 (67%); of these, 94 (69%) occurred at residences.

Based on review of these forms by state and county health department and fire department personnel to determine opportunities for intervention, 55 (40%) of the 137 incidents were attributed to a lapse in supervision; 48 (35%), to absence of a pool fence (i.e., a fence that completely encloses the pool and isolates it from the house and play area); 19 (14%), to an inadequate or unclosed gate or latch; three (2%), to an inadequate fence; and 12 (9%), to other causes.

The proportion of drownings and near drownings considered preventable by a pool fence was higher during the colder months (October through April, 29 [56%] of 52 drownings and near drownings) than during hotter months (May through September, 19 [22%] of 85).

Substantial morbidity and mortality also occurred among persons who were admitted to hospitals for near drowning. Of 398 children admitted to a major children's hospital in the state from July 1982 through July 1989 for near drownings, 74 (19%) died, and 36 (9%) were discharged as neurologically impaired (Phoenix Children's Hospital, unpublished data, 1989).

Reported by: TJ Flood, MD, M Aickin, PhD, Div of Disease Prevention, SJ Englender, MD, State Epidemiologist, Arizona Dept of Health Svcs; D Tucker, Phoenix Fire Dept, Phoenix, Arizona. Unintentional Injuries Section, Epidemiology Br, Div of Injury Control, Center for Environmental Health and Injury Control, CDC.

Editorial Note: Factors possibly associated with the increased risk for child drowning and near drowning in Arizona include the state's numerous swimming pools, relatively higher temperatures, and relatively longer outdoor swimming season.

---

*Arizona uses the following *International Classification of Diseases, Ninth Revision*, rubrics to define child drowning: E830, E832, E910, E984.
†In this report, near drowning is defined as a life-threatening incident in which the child was apneic or pulled from under the surface of the water. Outcomes of near-drowning incidents were not tracked for the Maricopa County study; incidents in which the child was struggling or both floating and breathing when rescued were not counted as near-drowning incidents.

Reports from Australia and New Zealand suggest that pool fencing alone could substantially reduce childhood drownings in pools in those countries (*2,3*). Data from Maricopa County suggest that pool fencing, in combination with adequate gates and latches, could have prevented 70 (51%) of the 137 drownings or near drownings reported. Because 40% of the incidents were attributed to a lapse in supervision (i.e., the supervisor's attention was diverted or a child was momentarily unobserved while the adult performed a chore in the pool area), educating parents about constant vigilance at a pool should complement an emphasis on passive barriers to the pool. To reduce the higher proportion of deaths preventable by pool fences in winter months, when supervision tends to decrease around the pool environment, education should emphasize the need to maintain vigilance if the pool is not drained.

Measures to reduce childhood drownings and near drownings in Maricopa County have included mandatory fencing and barriers around swimming pools and educational campaigns conducted by Maricopa County fire departments to increase the public's awareness of child safety relating to water recreation. Other measures have included instruction on the maintenance of gates and latches, cardiopulmonary resuscitation classes, and requests of the swimming pool and home building industries to improve the design and placement of pools.

References
1. CDC. Childhood injuries in the United States. Am J Dis Child 1990;144:627–46.
2. Langley J. Fencing of private swimming pools in New Zealand. Community Health Stud 1983;7:285–9.
3. Pearn J, Nixon J. Prevention of childhood drowning accidents. Med J Aust 1977;1:616–8.

Diving-Associated Spinal Cord Injuries During Drought Conditions — Wisconsin, 1988

As many as 1,000 spinal cord injuries occur each year in the United States when persons—predominately males aged 15–25 years—dive into swimming pools or natural bodies of water. Strategies to prevent diving-associated spinal cord injuries include conducting public education and poster campaigns, posting warnings in areas that are hazardous for diving, and encouraging divers to determine the depth of the water before diving by wading or jumping into the water feet first.

—MMWR Vol. 37/No. 30, August 5, 1988, pp. 453–4

Diving-Associated Spinal Cord Injuries During Drought Conditions — Wisconsin, 1988

From June 1 through July 15, 1988, eight patients with cervical spinal cord injuries (SCIs) that occurred from diving into water were reported to two spinal injury centers in Milwaukee, Wisconsin. During similar periods in 1986 and 1987, five and three such injuries, respectively, were reported to these centers.

The injured persons ranged in age from 15 to 23 years, and all eight were male. One was injured in a swimming pool and is not included in this report. The other seven were injured in natural bodies of water, and six of the seven were familiar with these bodies of water. All patients believed the water was deeper than it actually was. Five patients have some degree of quadriplegia with or without fracture (Table 1), and two have either no neurologic deficits or no residual neurologic deficits.

Wisconsin, like other states in the Midwest and Southeast, has experienced drought conditions. This year's rainfall has averaged about 6 inches below that of last year for these regions. Water levels in inland lakes are between 10 inches and 10 feet below normal levels.

TABLE 1. Selected characteristics of seven patients referred to two spinal injury centers for non-swimming-pool diving-related injuries — Milwaukee, Wisconsin, June 1–July 15, 1988

Age (years)	Body of water	Anatomic site of injury*	Resulting injury
18	lagoon	C7	quadriplegia
18	river or pond	C6	quadriplegia
19	lake	C6	fracture, no residual neurologic deficits
22	lake	C7	quadriplegia
22	lake	C6	fracture, no residual neurologic deficits
23	lake	C7	incomplete quadriplegia
23	lake	C7	incomplete quadriplegia

*C = cervical spine.

Reported by: DJ Maiman, MD, Veterans Administration Hospital, Milwaukee; D Kunelius, Wisconsin Dept of Natural Resources; H Weiss, MPH, HA Anderson, MD, JP Davis, MD, State Epidemiologist, Wisconsin Dept of Health and Social Svcs. Div of Field Svcs, Epidemiology Program Office; Div of Injury Epidemiology and Control, Center for Environmental Health and Injury Control, CDC.

Editorial Note: Each year, 10,000–20,000 new SCIs occur in the United States (1). As many as 1,000 of these injuries result when persons—predominantly males aged 15–25 years—dive into swimming pools or natural bodies of water (1,2). In a 1970–1971 case series in California, 15 cases of quadriplegia were reported. One resulted from a dive into a swimming pool; the other 14 cases resulted from dives into rivers, streams, lakes, or oceans (3). Only three of these injured persons from California had objective evidence of the depth of the water at the time of injury; most of the divers had underestimated it.

This summer's drought, affecting most midwestern and many southern states, has resulted in record-low water levels in rivers, lakes, and streams. These conditions probably increase the risk of SCIs from diving, even in natural bodies of water previously considered safe. Because of extremely low water levels, no one should dive—even into a familiar body of water—until the depth of the water has been objectively measured.

Several strategies to prevent diving-associated SCIs have been suggested. States can closely monitor water levels in natural bodies of water during periods of low rainfall and can post warning signs to alert potential divers of hazards. In some localities, public education and poster campaigns have been used, and areas that are too shallow for diving have been posted as being hazardous. Other strategies urge divers to determine the depth of the water by wading into it before diving or by first jumping feet first into the water (4).

In 1987, the Council of State and Territorial Epidemiologists recommended that traumatic SCIs be designated as reportable injuries (5). Strengthening state-based surveillance of SCIs will help identify hazardous diving conditions under which SCIs may be more likely to occur. Surveillance can also assist in implementing and evaluating measures to prevent SCIs.

References
1. Kraus JF. Epidemiological aspects of acute spinal cord injury: a review of incidence, prevalence, causes, and outcome. In: Becker DP, Povlishock JT, eds. Central nervous system trauma status report—1985. Bethesda, Maryland: National Institute of Neurological and Communicative Disorders and Stroke, National Institutes of Health, 1985:313–22.
2. National Coordinating Council on Spinal Cord Injury. Head and spinal cord injury prevention. NCCSCI Dialogue 1988;(July):3.
3. Kewalramani LS, Kraus JF. Acute spinal-cord lesions from diving—epidemiological and clinical features. West J Med 1977;126:353–61.
4. Pierson P, Pierson E, Gelber B. A spinal cord injury prevention program. Nebr Med J 1986;71:133.
5. CDC. Acute traumatic spinal cord injury surveillance—United States, 1987. MMWR 1988; 37:285–6.

Drownings in the United States, 1978–1984

Drowning rates in the U.S. population have decreased modestly since 1978. Between 1978 and 1984, children <5 years old and young adults aged 15–24 years had the highest rates. Rates were highest in the South and lowest in the Northeast. Approximately 50% of drownings among teenagers and adults were alcohol-related.

—MMWR Vol. 37/No. SS-1, February 1988, pp. 27–33

Drownings in the United States, 1978–1984

Jama A. Gulaid, Ph.D., M.P.H.
Richard W. Sattin, M.D.
Division of Injury Epidemiology and Control
Center for Environmental Health and Injury Control

Introduction

Drowning is the third leading cause of injury deaths, surpassed only by motor vehicle- and fall-related deaths. It is also the second leading cause of injury deaths for persons ages 5-44 years (*1*). The U.S. Department of Health and Human Services set a national objective to reduce the crude death rate for drowning from 3.2/100,000 persons in 1978, the baseline year, to 1.5/100,000 persons in 1990 (*2*).

The purpose of this summary is to 1) describe the epidemiology of drowning in the United States, 2) review progress made since 1978 toward the 1990 objective, 3) discuss factors affecting progress toward this objective, and 4) recommend measures that will help attain this objective.

Methods

Data used to determine the number of drownings in the United States for 1978-1984 were obtained from annual mortality tapes of the National Center for Health Statistics (NCHS). NCHS receives reports of all deaths of U.S. residents in the 50 states and the District of Columbia. Deaths are coded according to the International Classification of Diseases (ICD), Adapted—Eighth Revision for 1978 and Ninth Revision for 1979-1984.

In this summary, nonboat-related drownings are defined according to ICD with an underlying external cause of death coded as E910; boat-related drownings are those coded E830 and E832. Information in the NCHS mortality tapes includes age, sex, date of death, race (white, black, or other), state where death occurred, and decedent's state of residence.

U.S. population estimates from the Bureau of the Census for 1978-1984 were used to compute rates (*3*). These data for the United States and for each of the four NCHS regions (Northeast, Midwest, South, and West) were used to compute crude death rates for drownings per 100,000 population. Regional rates were based on the number of deaths that occurred in a region rather than on the number of deaths to residents of the region, because regional environmental factors might be important determinants of rates. In fact, rates calculated both ways were almost identical.

Results

Between 1978 and 1984, an average of 6,503 persons drowned each year (Table 1). The number of drowning deaths decreased from a high of 7,026 in 1978 to a low of 5,388 in 1984. The overall crude death rate from drowning dropped 28% between 1978 and 1984, from a high of 3.2 deaths/100,000 population to a low of 2.3. Much of this decrease occurred among whites ages 5-24 years, blacks ages 10-24 years, and others ages 19-44 years. The rate of drowning for males dropped 28% between 1978 and 1984, whereas the rate for females dropped 20%. For each of these years, the death rate was nearly four times greater for males than for females and two times greater for blacks than for whites. For 1984, the South continued to have the highest drowning rates (3.0 deaths/100,000 population), followed by the West (2.9

TABLE 1. Drownings and drowning rates, by sex, race, and region, United States, 1978-1984

	1978		1979		1980		1981		1982		1983		1984	
	No.	Rate*	No.	Rate	No.	Rate	No.	Rate	No.	Rate	No.	Rate	No.	Rate
Sex														
Male	5,875	5.4	5,779	5.3	6,121	5.5	5,335	4.8	5,294	4.7	5,342	4.7	4,420	3.9
Female	1,151	1.0	1,093	0.9	1,136	1.0	942	0.8	1,057	0.9	1,011	0.8	968	0.8
Race														
White	5,407	2.8	5,302	2.7	5,623	2.9	4,836	2.5	4,884	2.5	4,975	2.5	4,137	2.1
Black	1,415	5.5	1,370	5.2	1,429	5.3	1,254	4.6	1,254	4.5	1,171	4.2	1,048	3.7
Other	204	4.8	200	4.4	205	3.9	187	3.3	213	3.5	207	3.2	203	3.0
Region														
Northeast	836	1.7	839	1.7	911	1.9	763	1.6	771	1.6	779	1.6	710	1.4
Midwest	1,368	2.3	1,316	2.2	1,304	2.2	1,174	2.0	1,125	1.9	1,129	1.9	934	1.6
South	3,169	4.3	3,164	4.4	3,397	4.5	2,790	3.7	2,935	3.8	2,891	3.7	2,397	3.0
West	1,653	4.0	1,553	3.6	1,645	3.8	1,550	3.5	1,520	3.4	1,554	3.4	1,347	2.9
Total deaths	7,026	3.2	6,872	3.1	7,257	3.2	6,277	2.7	6,351	2.7	6,353	2.7	5,388	2.3

*Drownings/100,000 population.

deaths/100,000 population). The Northeast continued to have the lowest rates (1.4 deaths/100,000 population), and the overall death rate/100,000 population declined markedly, from 2.7 in 1983 to 2.3 in 1984.

The highest drowning rates occurred among children <5 years of age, especially among 2-year-olds (Figure 1). Rates generally declined with age; however, young adults ages 15-24 years also had high rates.

Drowning rates for blacks were consistently higher than those for whites except at ages 0-3 years. At these ages, white children had between 1 1/2 and 2 1/2 times the rate of black children. In the first six decades, other races had drowning rates between those of blacks and whites (Figure 2); however, after age 64, drowning death rates for other races were higher than those for blacks and whites. At ages ≥85, other races had the highest death rates of any age or racial group.

The number of drownings peaked in the summer (Figure 3). More than 50% of these deaths occurred from June through August; less than 10% occurred from December through February. Most drownings (about 82%) were not associated with boats (Table 2). Nonboat-related drowning rates were highest for blacks and lowest for whites. Boat-related drownings per 100,000 population were similar in the three racial groups, but remained lowest in whites except in 1980 and 1981, when the rates were lowest in other races.

Discussion

The overall drowning rates decreased modestly between 1980 and 1981, remained steady between 1981 and 1983, and declined in 1984. Children <5 years old and young adults ages 15-24 had the highest rates. For children <5 years old, whites had rates almost twice as high as those of blacks; for almost all other ages, drowning

FIGURE 1. Drowning rates, by age group, United States, 1978-1984

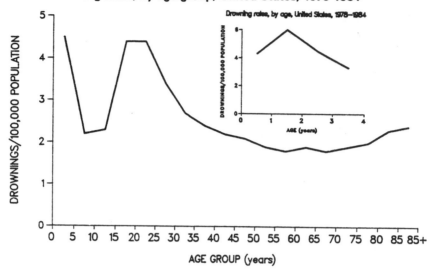

FIGURE 2. Drowning rates, by age group and race, United States, 1978-1984

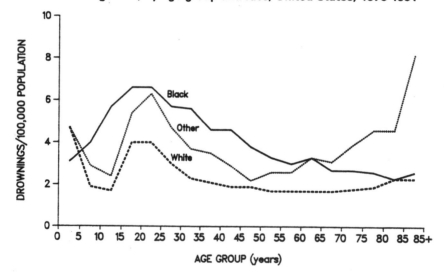

rates for blacks exceeded those for whites. The South had the highest drowning rates, and the Northeast had the lowest. The rates of boat-related drownings were slightly lower for whites than for other racial groups except in 1980 and 1981, and most of these drownings occurred in the summer.

Circumstances of drowning and the profile of a person who has drowned vary by age, race, and sex. For instance, swimming pools have been shown to present the

FIGURE 3. Distribution of drownings, by season, United States, 1978-1984

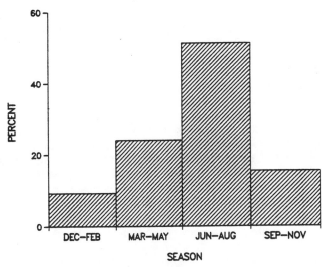

TABLE 2. Drownings and drowning rates, by cause and race, United States, 1978-1984

	1978		1979		1980		1981		1982		1983		1984	
	No.	Rate*	No.	Rate	No.	Rate	No.	Rate	No.	Rate	No.	Rate	No.	Rate
Boat-related														
Race														
White	1,026	0.5	1,000	0.5	1,013	0.5	878	0.4	882	0.4	923	0.5	768	0.4
Black	170	0.7	165	0.6	182	0.7	152	0.6	180	0.7	143	0.5	150	0.5
Other	46	1.1	29	0.6	19	0.4	14	0.2	31	0.5	33	0.5	26	0.4
Total	1,242	0.6	1,194	0.5	1,214	0.5	1,044	0.5	1,093	0.5	1,099	0.5	944	0.4
Nonboat-related														
Race														
White	4,381	2.3	4,302	2.2	4,610	2.4	3,958	2.0	4,002	2.0	4,052	2.0	3,369	1.7
Black	1,245	4.8	1,205	4.6	1,247	4.7	1,102	4.1	1,074	3.9	1,028	3.7	898	3.2
Other	158	3.7	171	3.8	186	3.5	173	3.0	182	3.0	174	2.7	177	2.6
Total	5,784	2.6	5,678	2.5	6,043	2.7	5,233	2.3	5,258	2.3	5,254	2.3	4,444	1.9

*Drownings/100,000 population.

greatest aquatic hazard for toddlers (4). This hazard is most evident in California, the state with the highest number of children's drownings in pools and spas (5). Diving in swimming pools also presents risks of spinal cord injuries and deaths (4), and bathtub drownings present hazards for children and for adults >70 (6,7). Although drownings are much less common among females than males, in one study bathtub drownings accounted for almost 29% of all drownings among females, a much larger percentage than among males (7). More males than females drown at other sites, such as in rivers and lakes. The boat-related drowning rate is highest among blacks; further research is needed to determine reasons for this increased risk.

Reasons for the increased risk of drowning among young males ages 15-24 are less clear than those among children. Evidence points to many complex human and environmental risk factors that include consumption of alcohol, nonuse of personal flotation devices (PFDs), poverty, climate, increased use of spas and hot tubs, inability to swim, and risks associated with the use of certain types of boats (4,5,8-10). An increased risk of drowning is associated with race; however, the increased risk among blacks and Native Americans may be associated with poverty, rural residence, and inability to swim (9). The variation in drowning rates for persons ages ≥49 years in the "other races" category may be due to the small number of persons who drown at these ages.

The high frequency of death in summer suggests that climate is a causative factor in drowning. Discomfort caused by summer heat probably leads to swimming in undesignated swimming areas, where about 80% of drownings occur (9). Although unquantified, the increased frequency and duration of exposure to water may explain the higher rates of drowning deaths in the summer; however, in areas with colder climates, such as Alaska, exposure to cold water may increase the risk of drowning (9). Most boat-related drownings occur in the summer. Data from the U.S. Coast Guard show that 82% of boat-related drownings in 1985 were associated with inappropriate PFDs or with the nonuse of PFDs. Open boats, small boats (<16 ft), and high-speed boats (≥75 hp) were most frequently involved in fatalities (10).

Several interventions have helped reduce the number of drownings. Adding a fence with latchgates to home pools has substantially reduced drownings in pools (11-13). For boat-related drownings, reasons for the decline in fatalities per 100,000 recreational boats (from 20.8/100,000 in 1979 to 6.9 in 1985) have not been determined. This decline, however, may be due to improvements in boat safety, regulations, increased use of PFDs, and—in cold climates—the use of lifesaving equipment suits (10).

Since approximately 50% of teenage and adult drownings are alcohol related (6,8), interventions concerning alcohol use and the restriction of alcohol use in boats may have an impact on drowning mortality. Research and health promotion initiatives continue to heighten public awareness of associations between alcohol abuse and adverse health effects, including injuries. Governmental and nongovernmental agencies responsible for these initiatives include the U.S. Coast Guard; the Alcohol, Drug Abuse, and Mental Health Administration, Public Health Service; the Center for Health Promotion and Education, CDC; and various state, community, private, and voluntary organizations.

Several limitations have led to an underestimated drowning rate in one instance and may have led to overestimated rates in another. The overall drowning rate is underestimated because the 1990 objective excludes drownings related to motor vehicles, suicides, and undetermined intentionality, which together account for about 1,500 deaths per year (*9*). Some regional rates may be slightly overestimated because computations were based on the number of deaths that occurred in states, which may include some deaths of nonresidents. Nevertheless, findings of this study were not measurably affected, since such large (regional) populations were used as denominators. Thus, the findings of this study provide a good estimate of drowning rates as delineated by the 1990 objective.

Overall, the 1990 objective is limited as an indicator of the public health impact of drowning because it uses crude death rates without addressing the importance of specific high-risk populations. For example, the objective of 1.5 deaths/100,000 persons is met for females and, overall, nearly met for adults ages 50-79. However, the objective is not met for males, blacks, other races, children <5 years old, or young adults ages 15-34. Future objectives should address the mortality and morbidity of the population. To monitor the impact of future interventions in achieving their objectives, injury surveillance systems should be strengthened or initiated where they do not exist. The only source of nationwide drowning information is NCHS, and data from that source are subject to an 18-month delay. Drowning surveillance at the state level can be based either on death certificates or on medical examiner/coroner data. Data from these sources are subject to fewer delays.

In conclusion, progress has been made since 1978, as shown by the decline in drowning rates in the U.S. population. Yet, much needs to be done if the projected rate, which is almost two-thirds the current rate of 2.3 deaths/100,000 persons, is to be achieved by 1990. Further reduction of aquatic deaths and injuries is possible, but this will require implementing intervention strategies such as those suggested by 25 leaders in injury control during a 1981 National Conference on Injury Control cosponsored by CDC (Appendix) (*4,14*). In addition, more research is needed before public health personnel can evaluate implemented strategies and unravel the complex human, technologic, and mechanical factors associated with drowning, especially for high-risk groups.

References
1. National Safety Council. Accident facts, 1985. Chicago: National Safety Council, 1986.
2. CDC. Mid-course review report for the 1990 injury prevention objectives. Atlanta, Georgia: CDC, 1985.
3. US Department of Commerce, Bureau of the Census. Current population estimates and projections. Washington, DC: US Department of Commerce. (Series P-25, nos. 917, 1982; 957, 1984; 998, 1986; and 1,000, 1987.)
4. CDC. Aquatic deaths and injuries—United States. MMWR 1982;31:417-9.
5. US Consumer Product Safety Commission, National Pool and Spa Institute. National pool and spa safety conference (report). Washington DC: US Consumer Product Safety Commission, 1985.
6. CDC. Drownings—Georgia, 1981-1983. MMWR 1985;34:281-3.
7. O'Carroll P. Drowning mortality in Los Angeles County, 1978-84. Presented at the APHA Meeting, Washington DC, November 20, 1985.
8. Dietz PE, Baker SP. Drowning epidemiology and prevention. Am J Public Health 1974;64:303-12.
9. Baker SP, O'Neill B, Karpf RS. The injury fact book. Lexington, Massachusetts: DC Heath, 1984:155-65.
10. US Coast Guard. Boating statistics, 1985. Technical report COMDITINST M16754.1g. Washington, DC: US Department of Transportation, 1986.

11. Pearn JH, Wong RYK, Brown J III, Ching Y-C, Bart R Jr, Hammar S. Drowning and near-drowning involving children: a five-year total population study from the city and county of Honolulu. Am J Public Health 1979;69:450-4.
12. Pearn J, Brown J III, Hsia EY. Swimming pool drownings and near-drownings involving children: a total population study from Hawaii. Milit Med 1980;145:15-8.
13. Milner N, Pearn J, Guard R. Will fenced pools save lives? a 10-year study from Mulgrave Shire, Queensland. Med J Aust 1980;2:510-1.
14. Teret SP, Baker SP, Trinkoff AM, DeFrancesco S, eds. Report of the National Conference on Injury Control (Johns Hopkins School of Hygiene and Public Health, May 18-19, 1981). Atlanta, Georgia: CDC, 1981.

Appendix

Selected Strategies of Intervention for Aquatic Deaths and Injuries

1. Develop and implement standards that govern safe pool design.
2. Require licensing for private and public pool construction and ownership based on certain safety requirements, including adequate fencing and accessible rescue and resuscitation equipment.
3. Require sign-posting in known hazardous-water areas regarding depth, undertow, or slippery banks.
4. Restrict the sale and consumption of alcoholic beverages in boating, pool, harbor, marina, and beach areas.
5. Impose sanctions for drunken boat drivers.
6. Integrate information into health department home-visit programs to make parents aware of pool, pond, and bathtub hazards.
7. Develop and institute programs for employees who work in or near bodies of water on how to recognize hazardous, environmental conditions and on emergency procedures that reduce the consequences of water-related injuries (e.g., procedures for extrication).
8. Conduct surveillance programs using emergency medical service logs, lifeguard data, coroners' records, and data from environmental groups, which are critical to evaluating the effectiveness of interventions.

Source: MMWR 1982;31:417-9.

Drownings at U.S. Army Corps of Engineers Recreation Facilities, 1986–1990

Most of the drownings included in this report occurred during swimming and wading (62% occurred outside designated swimming areas), boating activities, and fishing from shore. The Centers for Disease Control and Prevention recommends restricting swimming and wading to designated areas.

—MMWR Vol. 41/No. 19, May 15, 1992, pp. 331–3

Drownings at U.S. Army Corps of Engineers Recreation Facilities, 1986–1990

The U.S. Army Corps of Engineers, Department of the Army, is the largest federal provider of water-based recreation facilities in the United States. Each year, the Corps records more than 2.3 billion visitor hours at its 460 lakes and reservoirs and estimates that 25 million persons visit one of its facilities at least once each year (*1*). Since 1986, the Corps has promoted water safety through educational campaigns at its facilities nationwide. The Corps, in collaboration with CDC, reviewed information about drownings and water-safety activities for 1986 through 1990 to assist in improving its water-safety programs. This report summarizes the assessment and describes water-safety measures the Corps is implementing to prevent drownings and other injuries.

The Corps compiles data on all deaths that occur at Corps recreation facilities. Data reported by park managers include demographic characteristics and information on the circumstances and locations of deaths.

From 1986 through 1990, 1107 persons drowned at Corps facilities. Of these, 334 (30%) were aged 16–25 years, 140 (13%) were aged 26–30 years, and 65 (6%) were children aged ≤5 years. Most persons who drowned (981 [89%]) were males. More than half of the drownings (572 [52%]) occurred on Saturday or Sunday (Figure 1).

FIGURE 1. Number of drownings at U.S. Army Corps of Engineers recreation facilities, by day of week, 1986–1990

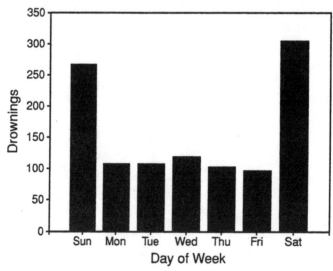

Rates of drowning (number per million visitor-days) were highest in 1986 (1.3) and lowest in 1988 (1.0); the death rate for drowning has remained stable after an initial decline in 1986.

For each year during 1986–1990, most drownings occurred during swimming and wading activities (488 [44%]), followed by boating activities (250 [23%]), and fishing from shore (187 [17%]) (Table 1). Of the swimming/wading-related drownings, 302 (62%) occurred outside the designated swimming areas.

TABLE 1. Number of drownings at U.S. Army Corps of Engineers recreation facilities, by activity and year, and rates per million visitor-days, 1986–1990

Category	1986	1987	1988	1989	1990	Total
Activity						
Swimming/Wading	136	98	92	71	91	**488**
Boating	55	65	41	38	51	**250**
Fishing from shore	44	38	33	38	34	**187**
Other	43	37	27	50	25	**182**
Total	278	238	193	197	201	1107
Million visitor-days	209	220	199	191	190	1010
Rate per million visitor-days	1.3	1.1	1.0	1.0	1.1	1.1

Each Corps facility has at least one designated swimming area, which employs buoys to prohibit boat and personal watercraft entry and signs and markers to inform swimmers of the limits of the designated zone. Designated swimming areas also are cleared of any trees, stumps, and debris and are constructed to achieve maximum depth and slope requirements, to improve swimming safety.

Since 1986, the Corps has promoted water safety nationwide through an annual, unified safety-education campaign, "Your Safety—Our Concern." This campaign has included audio and video tapes to be used as radio and television public service announcements and educational posters. In addition, the Corps uses permanent information and advisory posters at each facility to inform visitors to remain in designated swimming areas while swimming and wading.

Reported by: South Atlantic Div, U.S. Army Corps of Engineers, Atlanta. DW Hewitt, U.S. Army Corps of Engineers Headquarters, Washington, DC. Unintentional Injuries Section, Epidemiology Br, Div of Injury Control, National Center for Environmental Health and Injury Control, CDC.

Editorial Note: The findings in this report are consistent with patterns of drowning described previously for the United States. In particular, the rate of drowning is four times greater for males than for females, and drowning rates are highest for children aged <5 years and persons aged 15–24 years (2).

Through its national water-safety program, the Corps has emphasized preventing water-related fatalities at its facilities. By continuing to review and evaluate the causes for water-related deaths, all public and private recreational facilities can improve their water-safety efforts. Additional efforts the Corps can employ at its recreational facilities include 1) restricting swimming and wading to designated swimming areas; 2) engaging park managers to encourage visitors to restrict their swimming and wading to designated areas; 3) enhancing patrolling efforts at beach areas to ensure that visitors are swimming and wading safely; and 4) improving coordination with state agencies to foster more visibility of the enforcement of state boating laws. In

addition, the Corps' safety-awareness campaigns can address various topics including 1) warnings against alcohol consumption during water-based recreation activities
(e.g., swimming and boating), 2) promoting the use of personal flotation devices, and
3) warnings against swimming alone.

References
1. US Army Corps of Engineers. US Army Corps of Engineers Recreation Study: a plan prepared
   for the Assistant Secretary of the Army (Civil Works). Vol 1: Main report. Washington, DC: US
   Army Corps of Engineers, September 1990.
2. CDC. Drownings in the United States, 1978–1984. MMWR 1988;37(no. SS-1):27–33.

Drownings in a Private Lake — North Carolina, 1981–1990

Persons who swim in natural bodies of water may be at increased risk of drowning because of hazards including changing environmental conditions (e.g., depth, currents, and weather); insufficient warning signs; murky or cloudy water; close proximity to watercraft; and inaccessibility of emergency medical services.

—MMWR Vol. 41/No. 19, May 15, 1992, pp. 329–31

Drownings in a Private Lake — North Carolina, 1981–1990

Drowning is the third most common cause of death from unintentional injury in the United States (1); in 1989, in North Carolina, drownings were the leading cause of years of potential life lost before age 65 per death (2). From July 1 through August 31, 1990, two drownings occurred in a private lake in Beaufort County (1990 population: 42,283), North Carolina. A review of data from the Office of the Chief Medical Examiner (OCME) in North Carolina identified two additional drownings at this lake during 1981–1990, and a total of 17 drownings in the county during the 10-year period. At the request of the local health director, in October 1990, the North Carolina Department of Environment, Health, and Natural Resources (DEHNR) investigated the drownings using information from OCME files, hospital medical records, and ambulance reports. This report summarizes the investigation of the four drownings in the private lake, recommendations to prevent additional drownings, and characteristics of drownings in North Carolina in 1989.

This lake is on a private campground but is accessible to the general public. It is approximately 250 feet wide and 400 feet long with an average depth of approximately 9 feet, has a sandy bottom, and fills naturally by seepage of groundwater. To control algae, the owners had added a blue dye that made the water impermeable to light and reduced underwater visibility.

The decedents ranged in age from 7 to 15 years; all were male. Postmortem blood alcohol testing was obtained for three decedents; all tests were negative. Two decedents were reported by family members to be poor swimmers, and two were known to have been swimming without supervision. All the drownings occurred during June, July, or August; three were on a weekend or holiday, and all occurred between 1:30 p.m. and 4:30 p.m. Lifeguards were not present during any of the drownings, and a posted sign read "swim at your own risk."

All the drownings occurred in a heavily used part of the lake. Two persons had jumped off a diving board near the shoreline and reportedly never resurfaced. Another drowned approximately 8 feet from shore near the transition from shallow (approximately 4.5 feet) to deep (approximately 7 feet) water. The fourth drowned near a platform approximately 25–30 feet offshore. Two persons were under water ≤10 minutes and received cardiopulmonary resuscitation (CPR) at the scene. The other two were under water approximately 6 hours each. Three died at the scene, and the fourth survived 11 hours. None of these persons had external signs of trauma, and all drownings were determined to be unintentional.

Based on the investigation, during December 1990, state and local public health officials recommended that the owners of the lake implement the following measures: 1) maintain a lifeguard on duty during regularly scheduled hours of operation, 2) establish a safe-bather capacity based on a recommended amount of water surface per person, 3) display clearly labeled lifesaving equipment, 4) install float-lines marking water depths, 5) post signs displaying safety information, 6) use algae-control methods that do not reduce water clarity, and 7) consult a design engineer regarding the placement of recreational equipment at the site.

Owners of the lake had not acted on any of these recommendations by May 1991 when a fifth person (a 15-year-old boy) drowned at the lake. The county health director subsequently declared the lake to be an imminent hazard and instructed the owners to comply with several of the safety recommendations. As a consequence, by June 1991, the owners hired full-time lifeguards, restricted swimming in certain parts of the lake, posted depth markings, provided safety guidance for swimmers, and discontinued the use of coloring agents to control algae. No drownings have occurred at the lake since the owners implemented these safety recommendations. State and local health officials have continued to work with the owners of the lake to reduce drowning hazards and to evaluate the effectiveness of drowning-prevention actions.

To characterize drownings that occurred in natural swimming areas in North Carolina, the DEHNR reviewed data from the OCME, local health departments, and local police agencies for 1989 (the most recent year for which complete data were available). During 1989, 57 (38%) of the 151 drownings occurred in lakes or ponds. Of these 57 drownings, 32 (56%) occurred while the persons were swimming; in 10 of these incidents, the swimming area had been openly advertised as accessible for public swimming. However, six of these 10 incidents occurred in locations where lifeguards usually were not present.

Reported by: G Taylor, MPH, S Jones, Beaufort County Health Dept; D Brewster, TB Cole, MD, Injury Control Section, PD Morris, MD, B Williams, E Norman, MPH, Environmental Epidemiology Section, JB Butts, MD, Office of the Chief Medical Examiner, JN MacCormack, MD, State Epidemiologist, North Carolina Dept of Environment, Health, and Natural Resources. Div of Field Epidemiology, Epidemiology Program Office; Program Development and Implementation Br, and Epidemiology Br, Div of Injury Control, National Center for Environmental Health and Injury Control, CDC.

Editorial Note: In the United States, drowning rates are highest for males, children <5 years of age, and young adults 15–24 years of age (*3–5*). Factors commonly associated with drowning while swimming include lack of supervision (*6*); alcohol consumption (*7*); poor swimming ability (*7*); and absence of persons trained in lifesaving techniques, including CPR (*8,9*). Persons who swim in natural bodies of water may be at increased risk because of additional hazards including changing environmental conditions (e.g., depth, currents, and weather); insufficient warning signs; murky or cloudy water; close proximity to watercraft; and inaccessibility of emergency medical services.

In some states, laws have been enacted to establish basic safety requirements for natural swimming areas, including depth markings and warning signs, lifeguards, lifesaving equipment and first aid supplies, telephones for emergency use, safety plans, and restrictions on density (i.e., the number of persons allowed in a specified beach area). Further research is needed to evaluate the effectiveness of these drowning-prevention strategies. However, based on the results of the North Carolina investigation, states should strongly consider mandating basic safety requirements for natural swimming areas and discourage the use of algae-control methods that reduce water clarity.

References
1. CDC. Alcohol use and aquatic activities—Massachusetts, 1988. MMWR 1990;39:332–4.
2. Office of the Chief Medical Examiner, North Carolina Department of Environment, Health, and Natural Resources. North Carolina Medical Examiner System annual report, 1989. Raleigh, North Carolina: North Carolina Department of Environment, Health, and Natural Resources, 1990.
3. CDC. North Carolina drownings, 1980–1984. MMWR 1986;35:635–8.
4. CDC. Drownings—Georgia, 1981–1983. MMWR 1985;34:281–3.
5. CDC. Drownings in the United States, 1978–1984. MMWR 1988;37(no. SS-1):27–33.
6. Quan L, Gore EJ, Wentz K, et al. Ten-year study of pediatric drownings and near-drownings in King County, Washington: lessons in injury prevention. Pediatrics 1982;83:1035–40.

7. Dietz PE, Baker SP. Drowning—epidemiology and prevention. Am J Public Health 1974;64: 303–12.
8. Patetta MJ, Biddinger PW. Characteristics of drowning deaths in North Carolina. Public Health Rep 1989;103:406–11.
9. Wintemute GJ, Kraus JF, Teret SP, et al. Drowning in childhood and adolescence: a population-based study. Am J Public Health 1987;77:830–2.

North Carolina Drownings, 1980–1984

The North Carolina data support the hypothesis that persons with seizure disorders are at higher risk for drowning than the general population. They also support the need to increase public awareness of how alcohol use causes physical impairments that pose risks for swimmers, boaters, and fishermen.

—MMWR Vol. 35/No. 40, October 10, 1986, pp. 635–8

North Carolina Drownings, 1980–1984

Unintentional drownings in North Carolina in the period 1980-1984 were examined using records obtained from the North Carolina Office of the Chief Medical Examiner, which investigates all deaths from intentional and unintentional injury. A total of 1,052 persons drowned in the 5-year period, 953 of whom were North Carolina residents, for an average annual crude mortality rate of 3.2 drowning deaths/100,000 residents (Table 1).

Drowning rates per 100,000 population were higher for nonwhites than for whites (4.8 vs. 2.6) and higher for males than for females (5.8 vs. 0.8). Rates were highest for nonwhite males (8.8), followed by white males (4.7), nonwhite females (1.2), and white females (0.7) (Table 1). For all race/sex groups combined, drowning rates were highest for persons ages 15-29 years (4.6/100,000) (Table 2).

TABLE 1. Race- and sex-specific drowning rates and percentages of victims with blood alcohol concentrations ≥ 100 mg%, North Carolina, 1980-1984

| Race/sex of victims | Drownings* | | BAC ≥ 100 mg %[†] | |
	Number	Rate/100,000 residents	Number positive	Percentage positive
White male	521	4.7	154/474	32.5
White female	76	0.7	13/58	22.4
Nonwhite male	309	8.8	110/275	40.0
Nonwhite female	47	1.2	6/32	18.8
Total	953		283/839	33.7

*North Carolina residents.

[†]Of 1,052 drowning victims, 839 were tested for BAC.

TABLE 2. Age-specific drowning rates and percentages of victims with blood alcohol concentration ≥ 100 mg%, North Carolina, 1980-1984

| Age of victims (years) | Drownings* | | BAC ≥ 100 mg%[†] | |
	Number	Rate/100,000 residents	Number positive	Percentage positive
0-14	170	2.6	1/87	1.1
15-29	379	4.6	120/374	32.1
30-44	177	2.9	84/169	49.7
45-59	124	2.7	50/119	42.0
>60	103	2.3	28/90	31.1
Total	953		283/839	33.7

*North Carolina residents.

[†]Of 1,052 drowning victims, 839 were tested for BAC.

Most drownings occurred in lakes or ponds (39%), rivers or creeks (29%), or oceans and bays (11%). Six times as many drownings occurred in natural settings as in constructed facilities (e.g., bathtubs, pools).

At the time drownings occurred, most victims were swimming (41%) or fishing (15%) (Table 3). Drownings among members of certain demographic subgroups and among persons with some pre-existing medical conditions showed special associations with specific activities. For example, males accounted for 98% of all fishing deaths, and females accounted for 43% of all bath-associated deaths. White males accounted for a higher percentage (82%) of other recreational deaths (e.g., canoeing, sailing) than they did for all categories of drownings (56%). Children less than 5 years of age accounted for a higher percentage (25%) of bath-associated deaths than they did for all categories of drownings (6%). Although only 7% of all drowning victims were known to have seizure disorders, persons with seizure disorders accounted for 53% of all drownings resulting from bathing in a bathtub.

TABLE 3. Activity-specific percentages for drownings and percentages of victims with blood alcohol concentrations ≥ 100 mg%, North Carolina, 1980-1984

Activity involving victims	Drownings*		BAC ≥ 100 mg%[†]	
	Number	Percentage	Number positive	Percentage positive
Swimming	435	41.3	124/358	34.6
Fishing	157	14.9	42/137	30.7
Motor vehicle crash	83	7.9	35/69	50.7
Other recreation	65	6.2	15/52	28.8
Motorboating	51	4.8	14/40	35.0
Bath-associated	40	3.8	6/31	19.4
Rescue attempt	24	2.3	4/21	19.0
All other[§]	197	18.7	43/131	32.8
Total	1,052		283/839	33.7

*All drownings reported in North Carolina during 5-year period.
[†]Of 1,052 drowning victims, 839 were tested for BAC.
[§]Most activities involved unintentional entry into a body of water such as a creek, ditch, or pond.

Of all drownings, 56% were witnessed. However, the proportion of drownings that were witnessed ranged from 92% for swimming in a group to 3% for bathing in a bathtub. Of the 74 children ages 0-5 years who drowned, 59 (80%) were unattended. Of all persons who drowned, 2% drowned while attempting to rescue other drowning persons.

Blood-alcohol tests were performed for 839 (80%) of the 1,052 drowning victims. Alcohol was detected in 48% of victims tested; in 34% of victims tested, blood-alcohol levels were ≥ 100 mg%,* the legal level of intoxication in North Carolina. Blood-alcohol presence varied by demographic subgroup and predominated among nonwhite males (40%) and 30- to 44-year-olds (50%) (Tables 1 and 2).

Reported by M Patetta, MA, State Center for Health Statistics, P Biddinger, MD, Office of the Chief Medical Examiner, J Freeman, DVM, MPH, Environmental Epidemiology Branch, JN MacCormack, MD, State Epidemiologist, North Carolina Division of Health Services; Division of Field Services, Epidemiology Program Office, Division of Injury Epidemiology and Control, Center for Environmental Health, CDC.

Editorial Note: Drowning is the third most common cause of unintentional injury death in the United States (2). Drowning rates reported for North Carolina are higher than the overall national drowning rate of 2.4/100,000 population (1,2). Although most surveys of drowning consist of data derived from death certificate ICD codes, the North Carolina data reported here were abstracted from medical examiner reports, which also include findings of an investigation by a county medical examiner, autopsy reports, and toxicologic studies.

Age, race, and sex groups at highest risk for drowning in North Carolina are similar to those reported in national data (1). The proportions of North Carolina drownings occurring in lakes/ponds and rivers/creeks are similar to those reported for Georgia (3); however, the oc-

*The level of alcohol in the blood is defined as "milligrams of alcohol per 100 milliliters of blood" and is expressed as milligrams percent (mg%).

currence of drownings in natural settings relative to those in constructed facilities is proportionately higher. The proportions of drownings resulting from activities such as swimming and fishing (sometimes reported in other studies as "falling off docks or bridges") are similar to those reported from national surveys (2) and from other states (3,4).

Studies based on death certificates generally do not permit assessment of the impact of pre-existing medical conditions on drowning occurrence, because such information may not be provided in death certificates. The North Carolina data support the hypothesis that persons with seizure disorders are at higher risk for drowning than the general population (4,5); persons with seizure disorders are more likely to have a seizure following alcohol intoxication (6,7).

Because approaches to limiting the consumption of alcohol may be difficult to enforce, efforts should be made to increase public awareness of the physical impairments resulting from alcohol use which pose risks for swimmers, fishermen, and boaters. Strategies for injury prevention rely primarily on elimination of the hazard, creation of barriers between the hazard and the person at risk, instruction in personal protective measures against the hazard, and institution of measures to minimize damage associated with the hazard (8). In addition to human behavioral factors, intervention should focus on the modification of factors in the socioeconomic environment, as well as such factors as vehicles and equipment in the physical environment. Previous studies showed that alcohol was associated with about 50% of drownings among teenagers and adults (4). Enforcing limitations on the consumption of alcohol near water is difficult, although public awareness that the physical impairment resulting from alcohol use is as dangerous for swimmers, fishermen, and boaters as it is for motor vehicle operators could almost certainly be improved. Additionally, it must be realized that alcohol consumption among some high-risk individuals (e.g., 15- to 24-year-olds) is highly affected by the accessibility of alcohol. Sales and consumption of alcohol among this group are inversely related to the cost of alcohol (9). Recent upward alterations in the legal drinking age may lead to reductions in mortality associated with drowning.

Seventy-nine percent of North Carolina drowning deaths occurred in such natural settings as lakes, rivers, and bays. Of the 7,000 unintentional drownings that occur each year in the United States, about 17% involve boats—primarily recreational craft (3). Despite a 59% increase in the number of recreational craft in operation in the United States between 1973 and 1982, the recreational boating fatality rate (about 90% due to drownings) decreased 56% during the same period (3). Although the causes for this decrease have not been determined, they may include industry and government initiatives that have resulted in safety improvement in boats, increased use of personal flotation devices, and regulations that promote safe boating. Water safety instruction should be designed to lead to improvements in swimming ability, discourage risk-taking behavior such as alcohol use near water, encourage the use of personal flotation devices on boats, and teach rescue techniques that do not endanger the life of the rescuer. However, studies of the efficacy of water safety instruction programs are needed before such instruction is advocated as an effective intervention technique (10).

Although most North Carolina drownings do not occur in settings—such as pools—that could be fenced or drained when not in use, in the United States as a whole, most home-related drownings do occur in swimming pools and bathtubs. Therefore, child-proof fencing with self-latching gates around potentially dangerous bodies of water, including swimming pools, may reduce drowning among young children (11).

References
1. Baker, SP, O'Neill B, Karpf RS. The injury fact book. Lexington, Massachusetts: Lexington Books, 1984.
2. National Safety Council. Accidents facts, 1985. Chicago, Illinois: National Safety Council, 1985.
3. CDC. Drownings—Georgia, 1981-1983. MMWR 1985;34:281-3.
4. Dietz PE, Baker SP. Drowning: epidemiology and prevention. Am J Public Health 1974;64:303-12.
5. Greensher J. Prevention of childhood injuries. Pediatrics 1984;74:970-5.
6. Pearn J. Drowning and alcohol. Med J Aust 1984;141:6-7.
7. Plueckhahn VD. Alcohol and accidental drowning. A 25-year study. Med J Aust 1984;141:22-5.
8. Robertson LS. Injuries—causes, control strategies, and public policy. Lexington, Massachusetts: Lexington Books, 1983.
9. Mosher JF, Beauchamp DE. Justifying alcohol taxes to public officials. J Public Health Policy 1983 (December):422-39.
10. Waller JA. Injury control—a guide to the causes and prevention of trauma. Lexington, Massachusetts: Lexington Books, 1985.
11. Hearn JH, Wong RYK, Brown J, et al. Drowning and near-drowning involving children: a five-year total population study from the city and county of Honolulu. Am J Pub Health 1979;69:450-4.

Suction-Drain Injury in a Public Wading Pool — North Carolina, 1991

A child may be severely injured within seconds after sitting on a suction drain in a swimming or wading pool. Injuries can be prevented through interventions that prevent vacuums from forming when the suction-drain vents are covered. Interventions include antivortex covers or grates installed over the drains.

—MMWR Vol. 41/No. 19, May 15, 1992, pp. 333–5

Suction-Drain Injury in a Public Wading Pool —
North Carolina, 1991

On June 16, 1991, a 3-year-old girl playing in a public wading pool sat on the pool's uncapped suction drain. The child appeared to be stuck on the drain, and the pool attendant quickly turned off the pool's suction pump. As a consequence of sitting on the drain, the child sustained severe internal injuries requiring surgical repair. This report summarizes the investigation of this incident by the North Carolina Department of Environment, Health, and Natural Resources (DEHNR) and describes safety measures to prevent injuries among children caused by pool suction drains.

Following the episode at the wading pool, the child was examined at a hospital and had perianal bruising and prolapse of the rectal mucosa. The prolapse was manually reduced, and a pelvic computerized tomography scan showed no evidence of a rectal leak; however, by June 17, she had evidence of localized peritonitis. An exploratory laparotomy revealed a long anterior laceration of the seromuscular layer of the rectosigmoid colon; the mucosal tube was intact but ischemic and was separated circumferentially from the outer layers of the bowel wall. The laceration was repaired and a sigmoid colostomy performed.

The investigation by the DEHNR revealed that the wading pool where this injury occurred had a three-quarter–horsepower suction pump that was not linked to the adjacent adult pool or any other outlet. At the time of the injury, the antivortex drain cover that had previously covered the drain had been removed. Since the incident, the antivortex drain cover has been secured to the drain to prevent further suction injuries.

Reported by: NA Shorter, MD, Section of Pediatric Surgery, Duke Univ Medical Center, Durham; JP Woodell, Durham County Health Dept; TB Cole, MD, Injury Control Section, JA Hayes, MSPH, Div of Environmental Health, JN MacCormack, State Epidemiologist, North Carolina Dept of Environment, Health, and Natural Resources. Unintentional Injuries Section, Epidemiology Br, Div of Injury Control, National Center for Environmental Health and Injury Control, CDC.

Editorial Note: The findings in this investigation are consistent with those from previous reports of abdominal injuries among children who sit directly on uncovered openings or vents capable of forming a strong vacuum when covered (1). When a child sits on an unprotected suction-drain vent, the child's perineum can form a firm seal that creates a vacuum capable of relaxing the anal sphincter. This negative pressure on the exposed rectal walls can result in prolapse or intussusception; this, in turn, usually produces a full-thickness anterior bowel tear, creating the potential for evisceration of the mobile small intestine through the laceration and the anal canal. Damage to the mesentery can produce extensive irreversible small bowel ischemia requiring resection.

Since May 1, 1991, North Carolina has required all newly constructed public wading pools to be equipped with a surface skimmer and with interconnected double drains to prevent suction-drain injuries. However, pools constructed before May 1, 1991, have been allowed to continue operating with a single drain. The public pool involved in this incident was built before the standards became effective; however, the pool had been inspected 12 months before the injury occurred and had had an antisuction cover in place over the drain opening at that time.

Because a child may be injured within seconds of sitting on a drain, adult supervision alone does not effectively prevent suction-drain injuries. Suction-drain injuries can be prevented through interventions that prevent vacuums from forming when the vents are covered. Existing pools that may have a single suction-drain or multiple suction-drains that can be isolated by valves should be equipped with antivortex covers or with grates at least 12 inches by 12 inches over the drains to prevent the possibility of a vacuum forming if a child sits on a suction-drain opening (2). In addition, standards of the American National Standards Institute/National Spa and Pool Institute and the American Public Health Association specify that drain covers be secured in a way to prevent removal without special tools (2,3). Also, maintenance personnel should routinely inspect pool drains to ensure covers remain secure. Pools should not be operated if a suction-drain cover is missing, broken, or inadequately secured (2).

For new pools, water circulation systems should be constructed so that suction pumps are linked with more than one drain outlet; for example, the pump may draw water from two drains in the deepest part of the pool or from one drain and a surface skimmer, thus preventing a tight seal from forming if one drain is covered. In addition to these barriers, water-safety instruction courses should include specific instructions on the prevention of injuries involving pool equipment.

References
1. Cain WS, Howell CG, Ziegler MM, Finley AJ, Asch MJ, Grant JP. Rectosigmoid perforation and intestinal evisceration from transanal suction. J Pediatr Surg 1983;18:10–3.
2. National Spa and Pool Institute. American national standard for public swimming pools. Alexandria, Virginia: American National Standards Institute, National Spa and Pool Institute, 1991; publication no. ANSI/NSPI-1 1991.
3. American Public Health Association. Public swimming pools: recommended regulations for design and construction, operation and maintenance. Washington, DC: American Public Health Association, 1981:16–7.

Fatality at a Waterslide Amusement Park — Utah

This report of the death of a 13-year-old boy supports the need for safely designed drainage and recirculation systems not only at waterslide amusement parks but also in swimming pools and hot tubs. Drainage and recirculation pipes must be adequately covered at all times and small enough in diameter to prevent entrapment. State and local authorities should adopt safety standards to prevent injuries caused by entrapment at such facilities.

—MMWR Vol. 35/No. 26, July 4, 1986, pp. 429–30

Fatality at a Waterslide Amusement Park — Utah

On August 16, 1985, a 14-year-old male, his younger brother, and two friends went swimming at a large waterslide amusement park in Ogden, Utah. The children were playing in one of the slide-receiving pools (splash pool) where the depth was 4 feet. The 14-year-old (weight 134 lbs. [61.0 kg.], height 5 ft., 2 in. [1.59 meters]) was hanging onto the pool edge, dangling his feet over the submerged opening of the middle of three drain pipes, when he let go and disappeared into the pipe. Once inside the pipe, he was carried horizontally 93 feet, where he lodged in a 90-degree vertical bend inside the pumphouse (Figure 1). After 15 minutes, he was located, but resuscitation attempts were unsuccessful. An autopsy determined the cause of death as drowning.

FIGURE 1. Schematic of splash-pool drain pipe at waterslide amusement park where fatality occurred — Utah, August, 16, 1985

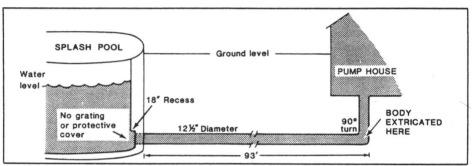

The waterslide park was constructed in 1984. Water from all six slides in the park drained into the splash pool where the boy was playing. The water then traveled by gravity through the three 12½-inch diameter polyvinyl pipes to a pumphouse where it was pumped to the top of the slides. The pipes were located in the side of the pool beneath a recessed overhang. Park employees reported that the cast iron grates covering the pipe inlets repeatedly fell off during the early part of the summer of 1985 because the cement eroded and, thus, was inadequate for holding the anchoring screws. As a result, the grates were removed. There were no other design features of the drainage system to prevent entry into the pipes.

Lifeguards were on duty at the time of the incident. The park was the seventh waterslide park designed by a company in Washington State, and its design met all local and state standards at the date of its opening in 1984. However, the park performed no routine checks of safety items.

An investigation of the death was led by the Weber-Morgan District Health Department, which had the statutory responsibility under Utah Code to "identify injury problems and develop standards for the correction and prevention of future occurrences." The final health department recommendations were (1) any drainage pipe with a diameter greater than 6 inches must have protective grating and backup entrapment prevention features that are approved by the health department before installation; (2) grates must be attached by a corrosive-resistant, secure anchoring system and must be attached so they cannot be removed by bathers; and (3) there must be a written record documenting monitoring of pool safety features.

Reported by M Nichols, MD, C Heninger, R Schwartz, O Orton, Weber-Morgan District Health Dept, S Patterson, Building Inspection, S VanderHeide, Sheriff's Dept, V Gabrenas, Attorney's Office, Weber County, F Jackson, Utah Dept of Health; H Walters, Intermountain Region, US Forest Svc; Div of Injury Epidemiology and Control, Center for Environmental Health, CDC.

Editorial Note: According to the U.S. Consumer Product Safety Commission (CPSC), this is the third reported death associated with a waterslide amusement park. The first death reported to the CPSC occurred in 1980 and was similar to that reported here: a 13-year-old male became entrapped in an 8-inch by 24-inch pool drain. The other reported fatality was a 35-year-old male who fell off a corkscrew turn in a waterslide.

In most waterslide splash pools, the drainage pipe inlet is too small to allow entrapment. Because six slides were installed, a large volume of water was recirculated, and the pipes draining the Ogden waterslide were unusually large. A safer alternative design would be to have more pipes with smaller diameter.

This problem extends beyond waterslide amusement parks. Since 1983, CPSC has received 10 reports of serious injury and three reported deaths associated with swimming-pool or hot-tub drainage systems. All 13 reports involved children 14 years of age or younger. In six of these incidents, including all three fatalities, the cover to the drain pipe had been removed. In all 13 incidents, the suction holding the child against the drain pipe opening or entangling hair was the primary cause of injury.

Recirculation and drainage systems may remain a source of serious injuries or deaths unless operators ensure that all drainage or recirculation pipes are adequately covered at all times to prevent the possibility of entrapment. Also, adequate safety standards for the design and operation of recreational waterslides, spas and hot tubs, and swimming pools should be adopted by state and local authorities. These standards should focus in particular on proper design features to prevent injuries caused by entrapment.

Recreational Boating Fatalities — Ohio, 1983–1986

Sports and recreational injuries are an important source of serious injuries and death in the United States. Potential prevention efforts include 1) a procedure for licensing recreational boat operators, 2) completion of an approved boating safety course, 3) improved enforcement of current laws, 4) stiffer penalties for operating boats while under the influence of alcohol, and 5) courses in swimming and rescue procedures.

—MMWR Vol. 36/No. 21, June 5, 1987, pp. 321–4

Recreational Boating Fatalities — Ohio, 1983–1986

Currently, more than 60 million people engage in recreational (noncommercial) boating activities in the United States, compared with 45 million in 1975 (*1*). Because of the potential for death associated with the sport, the Ohio Department of Health reviewed data on recreational boating-related fatalities in Ohio for the 4-year period 1983-1986. Analysis was based on data from the Division of Watercraft's Boating Accident Reporting (BAR) system (*2*). This system requires the operator of a numbered vessel involved in a boating mishap (incident) to file a report if the incident results in: 1) loss of life, 2) personal injury requiring medical treatment beyond first aid, 3) complete loss of the vessel, or 4) damage to the vessel and other property exceeding $200.00. Only incidents resulting in loss of life were analyzed because reporting appeared to be most thorough for this category.

There were 107 recreational boating incidents resulting in 124 fatalities during the years 1983-1986. Twenty-six incidents were reported in 1983; 29, in 1984; 25, in 1985; and 27, in 1986. One hundred (93%) of these involved only one boat. The remaining seven were two-boat collisions involving more than one boat operator. For collisions, data were analyzed only for the operator of the boat in which the fatality occurred.

Most fatal incidents (69%) occurred on Friday, Saturday, or Sunday, and 73% occurred between June 1 and September 30 (Figure 1). Fatal incidents occurred most often during the afternoon and early evening (56% between noon and 8:00 p.m.), while 9% occurred between midnight and 4:00 a.m. Although fatal incidents occurred in 50 of Ohio's 88 counties during the 4-year period, 44 of 107 incidents (41%) occurred within the jurisdiction of the eight counties bordering Lake Erie.

FIGURE 1. Fatal boating incidents, by month — Ohio, 1983-1986

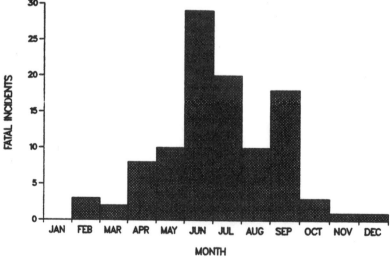

The boat operators involved ranged from 14 to 74 years of age; the mean age was 36.3 years. Operators had varied boating experience, but over 50% had >100 hours of experience on the water (Table 1). Alcohol use was noted in eight (7.5%) of the 107 reports. This information generally came from the investigating officials' reports and was based either on the testimony of witnesses or on direct physical evidence, such as the presence of alcoholic beverage containers. Confirmatory evidence, such as blood-alcohol levels, was usually not available.

TABLE 1. Recreational boating fatalities, by operator experience — Ohio, 1983-1986

	Fatal Events	
Operator Experience	No.	(%)
<20hrs.	21	(26.6)
20-100hrs.	16	(20.3)
101-500hrs.	19	(24.0)
>500hrs.	23	(29.1)
Unknown	28	—
Total	**107**	**(100.0)**

The greatest number of fatalities involved motorboats (Table 2). However, fatality rates were higher for incidents involving smaller boats, such as canoes and rowboats. The highest overall fatality rate was in the miscellaneous group, which includes inflatable boats and rafts, small plastic vessels, jet skis, houseboats or pontoon boats, and vessels not otherwise classified.

Nine different types of incidents led to fatalities. Capsizing accounted for 42% of them, and falls overboard accounted for 29%. Activities at the time of incident included cruising (38%), drifting (17%), and fishing (15%). One death was associated with water skiing, and none involved racing.

TABLE 2. Recreational boating fatalities, by type of boat — Ohio, 1983-1986

Boat Type	Registered Boats*	No. Fatal Incidents	No. Fatalities	Death Rate[†]
Motorboats (Open, Cabin, Sail)	983,600	60	70	7.1
Sail Only	86,018	4	5	5.8
Rowboats	89,647	13	13	14.5
Canoes/Kayaks	168,148	17	18	10.7
Miscellaneous	59,281	11	16	27.0
Unknown	—	2	2	—
Total	1,386,694	107	124	8.8 [§]

*Totals for 1983-1986.
[†]Per 100,000 registered boats.
[§]Death rate excludes fatalities for which type of boat involved was unknown.

Reported by: JK Hopewell, Div of Watercraft, Ohio Dept of Natural Resources; T Halpin, MD, MPH, State Epidemiologist, Ohio Dept of Health. Div of Field Svcs, Epidemiology Program Office; Div of Injury Epidemiology and Control, Center for Environmental Health, CDC.

Editorial Note: Sports and recreational injuries are an important source of serious injuries and death in the United States. Almost 90% of all recreational boating deaths result from drowning, with the remaining 10% attributable to falls, burns, and other causes (*3*). In 1983, approximately 1,100 drownings involved recreational boats (*4*). In 1985, 1,116 deaths were associated with recreational boats (*2*). With the intention of increasing the public's awareness of boating safety and available resources, the National Safe Boating Council* sponsors National Safe Boating Week each year. This year it is the week of June 7-13.

Studies suggest that boat-operator experience and courses on boating safety may reduce the risk of mishaps (*1,2*). In the Ohio study, nearly one-third of the operators reported <20 hours of boating experience. Neither boating courses nor boating experience, however, have been formally evaluated for their effectiveness in preventing boating mishaps and injuries.

Unlike motor-vehicle operators, recreational boaters are generally not required to be licensed, and many have received no formal training in boat operation and safety procedures (*5*). However, operators of recreational boats are required to be familiar with laws and regulations, and enforcement of these laws can play an important role in preventing boating injuries.

Previous reports have identified alcohol use as a major contributing factor to deaths associated with recreational boating (*1,3,5,6*). An estimated one-third to two-thirds of recreational boating fatalities each year may involve alcohol (*5*). The low rates of apparent alcohol involvement in Ohio (7.5%) may be due to underreporting. Since 1970, Ohio has prohibited anyone under the influence of alcohol from operating a vessel. The law was expanded in 1986 to permit enforcement officials to require blood-alcohol testing of boat operators if there are reasonable grounds to believe they are under the influence of alcohol. While most states have a law prohibiting persons under the influence of alcohol from operating a vessel, less than half of these laws define legal intoxication. In addition, enforcement of these laws varies from state to state. The Ohio law has not been evaluated for its effectiveness in reducing the number of deaths and incidents associated with alcohol use.

The U.S. Coast Guard, which is responsible for overseeing the BAR system, estimates that it receives reports on nearly all fatal boating incidents. However, it also estimates that <10% of nonfatal incidents are reported (*2*). Information contained in these reports is provided primarily by the boat operator and is supplemented by the investigating state or local official.

Because of limited data, this study did not evaluate information about the victim or about the operators and vessels not involved in fatalities. Ohio is one of the few states requiring registration of all watercraft. However, certain types of boats, such as canoes and rubber rafts, may be underregistered, and the recreational boating fatality rates may be disproportionately high for these.

Potential prevention efforts aimed toward reducing recreational boating mishaps and deaths include: 1) a licensing procedure for recreational boat operators similar to that for motor vehicle operators; 2) completion of an approved boating safety course prior to boat registration; 3) improved enforcement of current laws, such as those

---

*The U.S. Coast Guard has a toll-free Boating Safety Hotline: (800)368-5647. Information about National Safe Boating Week or the Council can be obtained by writing: Secretary, National Safe Boating Council, Inc., c/o Commandant (G-BBS-4), U.S. Coast Guard Headquarters, Washington, D.C. 20593.

restricting alcohol use and requiring personal flotation devices; 4) stiffer penalties for operating under the influence of alcohol; and 5) courses in swimming and rescue procedures.

References
1. Metropolitan Life Insurance Company. Recreational boating fatalities: 1978-82. Statistical Bulletin 1984;65(2):2-7.
2. U.S. Coast Guard. Boating statistics 1985. Washington, DC: US Department of Transportation, 1986; publication no. COMDTINST M16754.1G.
3. Baker SP, O'Neill B, Karpf RS. The injury fact book. Lexington, Massachusetts: Lexington Books, 1984.
4. National Safety Council. Accident facts. Chicago: National Safety Council, 1986.
5. Transportation Research Board. Proceedings of workshop on alcohol-related accidents in recreational boating. Washington, DC: National Academy of Sciences, National Research Council, 1986.
6. National Safety Council. Accident facts. Chicago: National Safety Council, 1984.

Softball Sliding Injuries — Michigan, 1986–1987

During the 2-year study period, 45 sliding injuries occurred on fields with stationary bases (medical charges, $1,223 per injury) compared with two such injuries on fields with break-away bases (medical charges, $350 per injury). The use of break-away bases in recreational softball leagues might provide a significant, cost-effective reduction in softball injuries from sliding.

—MMWR Vol. 37/No. 11, March 25, 1988, pp. 169–70

Softball Sliding Injuries — Michigan, 1986–1987

During the period 1986–1987, a study of the use of break-away bases to reduce sliding injuries was conducted in Ann Arbor, Michigan (1). The break-away base that was used in the study is anchored by rubber grommets to a rubber mat that is flush with the infield surface. The mat is anchored to the ground by a metal post similar to that used with standard stationary bases. Seven hundred foot-pounds of force, or one-fifth the force needed to dislodge a stationary base from its mooring, is required to release the break-away portion of the base.

The study evaluated injuries sustained during 633 games on two fields with break-away bases and 627 games on six fields with stationary bases. The players were college students, laborers, executives, physicians, and others ranging from 18 to 55 years of age. Players were assigned to one of four leagues on the basis of skill level and experience. Teams were assigned to playing fields on a random and rotating basis. All fields were maintained in the same manner.

All injuries requiring a player to leave the game were documented by the umpires. Local hospital emergency rooms, the University of Michigan Student Health Service, and private practice orthopedic surgeons were asked to keep logs of patients seen with softball-related injuries. All persons identified by these three surveillance systems were contacted to see whether their injuries had occurred while sliding. Patients who had been playing on the study fields were included in the analysis.

During the study period, there were 45 sliding injuries on the fields with stationary bases (7.2/100 games) and two sliding injuries on the fields with break-away bases (0.3/100 games) (rate ratio = 22.7; 95% confidence intervals, 5.6 to 71.4). Forty-three of the 45 injuries to players sliding into stationary bases involved the lead foot or hand. Twenty-four of the 45 injuries were ankle injuries; five were skin abrasions; five were knee injuries; three were finger fractures; and eight were from other causes. Medical charges for these 45 players were approximately $55,050 ($1,223/injury). The two injuries involving break-away bases comprised a nondisplaced medial malleolar ankle fracture and an ankle sprain. The total medical expense for these two players was approximately $700 ($350/injury).

Reported by: DH Janda, MD, EM Wojtys, MD, FM Hankin, MD, ME Benedict, MA, Univ of Michigan, Ann Arbor, Michigan. Epidemiology Br, Div of Injury Epidemiology and Control, Center for Environmental Health and Injury Control, CDC.

Editorial Note: In 1986, the National Electronic Injury Surveillance System of the U.S. Consumer Product Safety Commission estimated that 361,552 baseball-related injuries were treated in emergency rooms in the United States (2). This figure probably underestimates the actual number of injuries. The Amateur Softball Association of America estimates that 32 million individuals participate in softball leagues and that teams consist of an average of 15 persons and play approximately 22 games per year (unpublished data). Based on these data, it may be further estimated that about 23 million softball games are played annually in the United States.

Studies of recreational softball injuries have found that base sliding is responsible for 35% to 71% of injuries occurring during play, including abrasions, sprains, ligament strains, and fractures (3,4). These injuries are caused by the impact of rapid deceleration against stationary bases. Methods suggested to reduce base-sliding injuries have included prohibiting sliding, offering better instruction on sliding techniques, using recessed bases, and using quick-release bases (4,5). Prohibiting base sliding would be effective but might be met with resistance from some fans and participants. Holding instructional clinics on proper sliding techniques is a possibility for school-related organizations; however, this method might be impractical for community-based teams.

The prospective study in Michigan suggests that modifying the bases can alter the pattern and frequency of sliding injuries. If the stationary-base sliding injury rate of 7.2/100 games and the cost per injury of $1,223 reported in the study are representative, then approximately 1.7 million sliding injuries occur annually at a cost of over $2 billion. Similar calculations indicate that exclusive use of break-away bases would reduce injuries to just over 70,000 (a 96% reduction) and medical costs to $24 million (a 99% reduction).

The umpires indicated that break-away bases did not significantly delay play, even though sliding players dislodged the bases up to six times per game. Properly seated bases did not detach during routine base running, and the umpires did not have difficulty with judgment calls when the bases released. The bases were durable and easy to replace and lasted both seasons.

The use of break-away bases in recreational softball leagues might provide a significant, cost-effective reduction in softball injuries from sliding. However, injuries may still occur from runners' errors in judgment, improper sliding technique, poor timing, inadequate physical conditioning, and alcohol consumption.

References
1. Janda DH, Wojtys EM, Hankin FM, Benedict ME. Softball sliding injuries: a prospective study comparing standard and modified bases. JAMA 1988;259:1848-50.
2. US Consumer Product Safety Commission. The National Electronic Injury Surveillance System: January-December 1986. NEISS Data Highlights 1988;10.
3. Wheeler BR. Ankle fractures in slow-pitch softball: the Army experience. Milit Med 1987;152:626-8.
4. Janda DH, Hankin FM, Wojtys EM. Softball injuries: cost, cause and prevention. Am Fam Physician 1986;33:143-4.
5. Wheeler BR. Slow-pitch softball injuries. Am J Sports Med 1984;12:237-40.

Injuries Associated with Soccer Goalposts — United States, 1979–1993

The potential exists for serious injuries associated with improperly installed or used soccer goalposts. Accurately assessing the extent of such events and targeting prevention efforts requires calculating an injury rate through improved data collection.

—MMWR Vol. 43/No. 9, March 11, 1994, pp. 153–5

Injuries Associated with Soccer Goalposts — United States, 1979–1993

Injuries associated with sports can be related to a variety of factors, including participant's level of conditioning or training, failure to use safety equipment, contact, overexertion, difficulty in conducting the task required, mismatch in skill or size between players, and adverse environmental conditions. A rare but often fatal event is a blow caused by a falling soccer goalpost resulting from improper installation or use. From 1979 through 1993, 27 persons were injured or killed from falling soccer goalposts. This report describes three (two fatal) injuries associated with soccer goalposts and summarizes an analysis of all fatal and nonfatal soccer goalpost-related injuries reported in the United States to the Consumer Product Safety Commission (CPSC) during 1979–1993.

Case 1

A 16-year-old boy and two friends at a high school soccer field without adult supervision climbed the mobile soccer goalpost. As one person climbed on the horizontal header of the 600-pound steel goalpost, the goalpost tipped forward and struck the head of the 16-year-old, who was hanging from the header, and rendered him unconscious. Cardiopulmonary resuscitation at the scene and at the local emergency department was unsuccessful. He was pronounced dead 1 hour after the incident. An autopsy revealed severe blunt head trauma with multiple skull fractures and cerebral edema. Analysis of blood samples was negative for alcohol and drugs. The goalpost, which was commercially made and had been in service without incident for 6 years, was not anchored to the ground at the time of the incident.

Case 2

A 3-year-old boy was playing in front of a metal goalpost after a soccer game. As his father and brother were lifting one of the goalpost's corners to remove the net for storage, the goalpost fell, striking the boy's head and pinning him to the ground; he was rendered unconscious immediately. Cardiopulmonary resuscitation was unsuccessful, and the boy was pronounced dead approximately 1 hour later. The goalpost had not been anchored.

Case 3

A 9-year-old boy was playing goalie during a team practice when a wind gust blew over the unstaked steel soccer goalpost. The child tried to stop the fall of the goalpost when it struck his upper leg and fractured his femur. He was hospitalized for 6 weeks and disabled for 4 months before regaining useful leg function. The goalpost had been moved before the beginning of practice, and the seven steel stakes that secured it to the ground had been left behind.

Analysis of National Morbidity and Mortality Data

Data about persons injured or killed by falling soccer goalposts in the United States during 1979–1993 were identified by CPSC from 1) the National Electronic Injury Surveillance System (1) 2) newspaper clippings, 3) medical examiner reports, and 4) personal contacts made by soccer coaches or equipment manufacturers to CPSC. Each case was investigated through site inspections and interviews with the injured patient, a parent or other family member, a witness, and/or authorities responsible for purchase or maintenance of the soccer goalposts.

During 1979–1993, 27 injuries related to falling soccer goalposts were investigated by CPSC, of which 18 were fatal. Most (23) injuries occurred among males; the mean age of injured persons was 10 years. Head trauma was the principal cause of death in 14 of the fatal injuries and was diagnosed in two of the nonfatal ones.

Of the 27 goalposts involved, 26 were made of metal, usually steel or galvanized pipe; 23 of the goalposts were mobile, one was permanently installed, and three were of unknown type. Twenty-five injuries occurred when a goalpost fell forward, with the top crossbar striking the victim. Eighteen goalposts were not anchored, one was anchored poorly, and three were anchored properly; for five, the status could not be determined. Fifteen of the incidents occurred on a school field; 11, at a local or private field; and one, at an unspecified site. Four events occurred during a soccer game and four during practice; the remaining events occurred during times not involving games or practice. All 27 events were witnessed: in six cases, an adult was directly supervising and in visual contact with the victim; in eight, an adult supervisor was in the general vicinity, although not in visual contact. Four injuries were associated with a person climbing; seven, with a person swinging or doing chin-ups; six, with lifting the soccer goalpost; and four, with wind gusts. In 12 (nine fatal) incidents, the injured persons caused the goalposts to fall.

Reported by: J DeMarco, C Reeves, US Consumer Product Safety Commission. Div of Unintentional Injuries Prevention, National Center for Injury Prevention and Control, CDC.

Editorial Note: The findings in this report indicate the potential for serious injuries associated with improperly installed or used soccer goalposts. Regulation soccer goalposts can be manufactured from steel, aluminum, or metal pipe; measure approximately 8 feet by 24 feet; and weigh 250–800 pounds. Because the mouth of the goalpost is completely open to the playing field, only three sides are available for stabilizing the goalpost from forward falls. The reports to CPSC indicate that injuries typically result from climbing on goalposts, swinging or hanging from crossbars, or doing chin-ups on crossbars.

In the United States, soccer goalposts are manufactured by seven companies, and an undetermined number are produced by local machine shops without strict specifications. In 1990, CPSC issued a voluntary labeling standard for use of warning labels on the front and back of the crossbar and the front of the goalposts. Because of concerns about the inability of young children to read such warnings and the likelihood that older children would ignore these warnings, voluntary standards were adopted in 1992 by manufacturers; these standards specify the need to anchor or counterweight the goalposts using driving stakes, auger stakes, vertical pipe sleeves, or sandbags. If stakes are used, four are recommended—two on the rear and one on either side. Goalposts not in use should be chained to a fence or other permanent structure, placed goal-face down on the ground, or disassembled for storage. Additional information concerning these or other methods of anchoring is available from the Coalition to Promote Soccer Goal Safety, telephone (800) 527-7510 or (800) 531-4252.

The findings in this report demonstrate the potential benefit of using a national surveillance system to collect data on rare injury events. Accurately assessing the extent of such events and targeting prevention efforts requires calculating an injury rate through improved collection of numerator and denominator data and collecting exposure risk data (i.e., age and sex of injured person and level of competition). In addition, schools, park districts, and soccer associations should report injuries associated with falling soccer goalposts to the CPSC hotline, telephone (800) 638-2772. For injuries involving goalposts that were properly installed and used, specific information should be collected about the materials and method used to anchor these structures and soil and weather conditions on the day of the incident.

Reference
1. US Consumer Product Safety Commission. The NEISS sample: design and implementation. Washington, DC: US Consumer Product Safety Commission, March 1986.

Injuries Associated with Horseback Riding — United States, 1987 and 1988

During 1987 and 1988, an estimated 92,763 emergency room visits for horseback riding injuries were made. The majority of these injuries could have been prevented if horseback riders improved their safety practices. Such practices may be improved when horseback riders are trained by experienced instructors who 1) have successfully completed a horse-safety course from an accredited organization, 2) emphasize safe riding techniques, and 3) wear helmets while riding to set a good example for students.

—MMWR Vol. 39/No. 20, May 25, 1990, pp. 329–32

Injuries Associated with Horseback Riding — United States, 1987 and 1988

Each year in the United States, an estimated 30 million persons ride horses (*1*). The rate of serious injury per number of riding hours is estimated to be higher for horseback riders than for motorcyclists and automobile racers (*2*). The following report uses data from the National Electronic Injury Surveillance System (NEISS) to describe the epidemiology of horseback-riding–associated injuries in the United States during 1987 and 1988.

NEISS is an emergency-room based active injury surveillance program of the U.S. Consumer Products Safety Commission. NEISS records the most severe diagnosis listed on the emergency room record. Reports from NEISS can be used to develop national estimates of the number of persons with product-related injuries treated in hospital emergency rooms.*

During 1987 and 1988, an estimated 92,763 emergency room visits were made in the United States for injuries related to horseback riding. Although the greatest number of injuries occurred in the 25–44-year age group, injury rates were highest for 5–24-year-olds, especially for females (Table 1).

TABLE 1. Horseback-riding–associated injuries, by patient age and sex — United States, 1987 and 1988

Age (yrs)	Male		Female		Total		
	No.	Rate*	No.	Rate*	No.	(%)	Rate*
0–4	928	4.9	686	3.8	1,614	(1.7)	4.4
5–14	7,672	21.8	11,915	35.5	19,588	(21.1)	28.5
15–24	9,899	25.9	15,518	41.5	25,418	(27.4)	33.6
25–44	18,585	23.9	17,603	22.4	36,187	(39.0)	23.1
45–64	6,046	13.8	2,292	4.8	8,338	(9.0)	9.1
≥65	1,469	6.0	150	0.4	1,619	(1.7)	2.7
Total	44,599	18.7	48,164	19.2	92,763	(100.0)	19.0

*Rate for the 2-year period per 100,000 population.

Nearly half the injuries occurred at home or on a farm (Table 2). Soft tissue injury (e.g., laceration, contusion, or abrasion) was the most common diagnosis, followed by fracture or dislocation, strain or sprain, and concussion (Table 2). Most injuries to the extremities and trunk involved soft tissue, fractures and dislocations, and strains and sprains. Head and neck injuries were mainly soft tissue (56.9%), concussions (18.5%), and fractures or dislocations (11.0%). The 14,120 fractures to upper extremities represented the single most common site and type of injury.

Of the injured persons, 9.9% required hospitalization. More than two thirds of hospitalized persons had head and neck (42.2%) or trunk injuries (25.2%). The most common diagnoses for these patients were fractures or dislocations (55.1%) and concussions (17.2%).

---

*Sixty-two hospitals with emergency rooms located throughout the United States contributed to this data base each month in 1987, 61 contributed data from January through March 1988, and 62 provided data from April through December 1988. The NEISS code used for horseback riding injuries is product code 1239, "Horseback riding (activity, apparel, or equipment)."

TABLE 2. Emergency room visits for horseback-riding–associated injuries, by setting, diagnosis, and site — United States, 1987 and 1988

Characteristic	No.*	(%)
Place injured		
Home[†]	22,693	(24.5)
Farm[§]	19,232	(20.7)
Sports or recreation setting	13,195	(14.2)
Other property	8,612	(9.3)
Street	1,466	(1.6)
School	204	(0.2)
Unknown	27,363	(29.5)
Diagnosis		
Soft tissue[¶]	42,382	(45.7)
Fracture or dislocation	25,610	(27.6)
Strain or sprain	17,067	(18.4)
Concussion	3,249	(3.5)
Internal injury	1,953	(2.1)
Other**	2,504	(2.7)
Injury location		
Upper extremity	28,048	(30.2)
Lower extremity	21,631	(23.3)
Trunk	20,733	(22.4)
Head and neck	17,518	(18.9)
Multiple sites	4,835	(5.2)

*Numbers in each category may not total 92,763 because of rounding.
[†]Includes injuries occurring in a yard, garden, sidewalk, driveway, or farmhouse (not farm-related).
[§]Includes injuries occurring on farmland, pasture, forest, woods, barn, or other outbuilding.
[¶]Includes puncture wounds, hematomas, avulsions, contusions, abrasions, and lacerations.
**Includes 102 patients for whom the diagnosis was unknown.

Reported by: DB Hammett, MD, American Medical Equestrian Association, Waynesville, North Carolina. Unintentional Injuries Section, Epidemiology Br, Div of Injury Control, Center for Environmental Health and Injury Control, CDC.
Editorial Note: Estimates of the number of persons in the United States who ride horses each year are broad, and demographic data are unavailable. The lack of specific denominators for horseback riders requires the use of census data to determine rates. However, the rates in this report may inaccurately estimate the risks for injury. For example, one possible explanation for the higher rates in 5–24-year-olds is that persons in this group are more likely to ride horses.

The risks for severe injury to the head, trunk, abdomen, and pelvis associated with horseback riding are well defined (3–5). Although no national estimates exist for the number of fatal injuries associated with horseback riding, a review of state medical examiner records from 27 states for 1976–1987 identified 205 such deaths (6); head injuries were associated with more than 60% of these deaths.

Although falls account for most horseback-riding–associated injuries (*4,6*), in one study, fewer than 20% of riders had worn a helmet at the time of the fall (*3*). Even when riders wear headgear, the headgear may be decorative or improperly secured, thereby providing limited or no protection (*2,5,7*). Because of the potentially severe sequelae of head injury (*8,9*), horseback riders should wear a properly secured hard shell helmet lined with expanded polystyrene or similar material. Helmet use has been endorsed by several medical and trade organizations, and national performance standards for helmets are available (*10–13*).

Horseback riders can also be injured when they collide with fixed objects; are dragged along the ground with a foot caught in a stirrup; are crushed between the horse and ground; or are trampled, kicked, or bitten (*2*). Equipment problems associated with injuries include improper boot-stirrup fit; broken reins, bridles, or stirrup straps; and malfunctions of the stirrup-release mechanism (*2,10*).

To reduce injuries, riders should wear properly fitting heeled boots and nonskid gloves, avoid loose-fitting clothing, regularly maintain and inspect equipment, replace worn parts, and use appropriately sized stirrups (*2,10*). Safety practices of horseback riders may improve when they are trained by experienced instructors who have successfully completed a horse-safety course from an accredited organization, who emphasize safe riding techniques, and who themselves wear helmets while riding. In addition, riding safety may improve for riders who use appropriate techniques to stop, start, and turn a horse and to perform a rapid (emergency) dismount (*14*).

References

1. Bixby-Hammett DM. Accidents in equestrian sports. Am Fam Physician 1987;36:209–14.
2. Firth JL. Equestrian injuries. In: Schneider RC, Kennedy JC, Plant ML, eds. Sports injuries: mechanism, prevention, and treatment. Baltimore: Williams and Wilkins, 1985:431–9.
3. Grossman JA, Kulund DN, Miller CW, et al. Equestrian injuries: results of a prospective study. JAMA 1978;240:1881–2.
4. Gierup J, Larsson M, Lennquist S. Incidence and nature of horse-riding injuries: a one-year prospective study. Acta Chir Scand 1976;142:57–61.
5. Barber HM. Horseplay: survey of accidents and horses. Br J Med 1973;3:532–4.
6. Bixby-Hammett D, Brooks WH. Common injuries in horseback riding. Sports Med 1990; 9:36–47.
7. Mahaley MS, Seabar AV. Accident and safety considerations of horseback riding. In: Proceedings of 18th American Medical Association Conference on the Medical Aspects of Sports. Chicago: American Medical Association, 1976:37–45.
8. Kraus JF. Epidemiology of head injury. In: Cooper PR, ed. Head injury. 2nd ed. Baltimore: Williams and Wilkins, 1986:1–19.
9. Levin HS. Neurobehavioral sequelae of head injury. In: Cooper PR, ed. Head injury. 2nd ed. Baltimore: Williams and Wilkins, 1986:442–63.
10. Brooks WH, Bixby-Hammett DM. Prevention of neurologic injuries in equestrian sports. Physician Sports Med 1988;16:84–6,88,90,93–5.
11. Bixby-Hammett DM. Head injuries in the equestrian sports. Physician Sports Med 1983; 11:82–6.
12. National Highway Transportation Safety Administration. A report to Congress on the effect of motorcycle helmet use law repeal: a case for helmet use. Washington DC: US Department of Transportation, 1980; publication no. DOT HS 805-312.
13. American Society for Testing and Materials. Standard specification for headgear used in horse sports and horse-back riding (F1163-88). In: Annual book of ASTM standards. Philadelphia: American Society for Testing and Materials, 1988.
14. DeBenedette V. People and horses: the risks of riding. Physician Sports Med 1989;17:250–4.

Alcohol Use and Horseback-Riding-Associated Fatalities — North Carolina, 1979–1989

Horseback riding requires coordination, timing, and communication of physical signals between horse and rider. Alcohol use may impair equestrians by adversely affecting coordination and judgment and by lengthening reaction time.

—MMWR Vol. 41/No. 19, May 15, 1992, pp. 335, 341–2

Alcohol Use and Horseback-Riding-Associated Fatalities — North Carolina, 1979–1989

In the United States, an estimated 30 million persons ride horses each year (1). Total injury-related morbidity and mortality associated with horseback riding in the United States is unknown; however, during 1976–1987, 205 such fatalities occurred in 27 states (2). Even though alcohol use is a risk behavior for many types of injury, its role in horseback-riding–associated deaths has not yet been established. This report summarizes a study by the North Carolina Office of the Chief Medical Examiner (OCME) to characterize all horseback-riding–associated deaths during 1979–1989 and to determine what proportion of riders had used alcohol before death.

Thirty horseback-riding (including mule-riding)–associated deaths were identified; on average, one to three occurred each year. Sixteen (53%) decedents were male. Decedents' ages ranged from 7 to 68 years (median: 33.5 years).

Twenty-five persons were mounted on a horse at the time of the fatal event; four persons were trampled or kicked; and for one person, rider status was unknown. Twenty-one (70%) riders died when they fell or were thrown from the horse. Twenty (67%) riders died following head injuries (including one rider who drowned after striking his head, losing consciousness, and rolling into water); nine (30%) riders died from internal chest or abdominal injuries; and one rider drowned when he rode his horse into a lake.

Of 18 decedents tested for blood alcohol, six (33%) had detectable blood alcohol concentrations (BACs) of 0.6–3.6 g/dL (Table 1, page 341). Of 13 decedents who fell or were thrown from their horses, five (39%) had detectable BACs; none of the four decedents who were kicked or trampled had detectable BACs; and the rider who drowned had a BAC of 0.9 g/dL.

TABLE 1. Characteristics of fatal horseback-riding–associated injuries among decedents tested for blood alcohol concentrations (BACs) — North Carolina, 1979–1989

Yr. of injury	Age (yrs)	Sex	Mounted	Injury	Cause of injury	BAC (g/dL)
1982	27	M	Yes	Head injury	Thrown	Negative
1983	68	M	Yes	Head injury	Fell from mule	Negative
1983	23	M	Yes	Head injury	Fell from horse	Negative
1983	14	F	Yes	Abdominal injury	Horse and rider fell	Negative
1983	42	M	Yes	Drowning	Rode into lake	0.9
1984	30	M	Yes	Head injury	Fell from horse	3.6
1985	7	F	No	Head injury	Kicked	Negative
1985	26	F	Yes	Head injury	Thrown	0.6
1985	21	M	Yes	Head injury	Thrown	0.7
1986	43	M	Yes	Clavicle fracture with arterial avulsion	Thrown	Negative
1987	32	F	No	Liver laceration	Trampled	Negative
1988	61	M	No	Crushed chest	Trampled by wagon mule team	Negative
1988	15	F	Yes	Spinal hemorrhage	Fell from horse	Negative
1988	41	F	Yes	Head injury	Horse and rider fell	Negative
1989	7	F	No	Trunk injuries	Trampled	Negative
1989	46	F	Yes	Head injuries	Thrown	Negative
1989	34	M	Yes	Chest injuries	Thrown and trampled	3.1
1989	39	M	Yes	Abdominal injuries	Thrown	2.6

Reported by: DB Hammett, MD, American Medical Equestrian Association, Waynesville; TB Cole, MD, Injury Control Section, JD Butts, MD, Office of the Chief Medical Examiner, JN MacCormack, MD, State Epidemiologist, North Carolina Dept of Environment, Health, and Natural Resources. Unintentional Injuries Section, Epidemiology Br, Div of Injury Control, National Center for Environmental Health and Injury Control, CDC.

Editorial Note: Although estimates of the proportion of horseback-riding–associated injuries related to alcohol use have not previously been reported, the proportion of horseback-riding–associated deaths related to alcohol use in this report is similar to that for other unintentional injury-related deaths in North Carolina and in other locations. For example, in North Carolina during 1973–1983, alcohol was detected in 48.6% of all persons who died from unintentional injuries (including those caused by motor-vehicle crashes) and who were tested for alcohol as part of the OCME's system (3). In Sacramento, California, during 1967–1969, 37% of persons who died from falls and 26% of those who died from fire-related injuries had consumed alcohol before death (4).

The findings in this investigation are subject to at least two limitations. First, complete information on the circumstances of the fatal event (e.g., risk factors and use of protective equipment such as helmets) was not available. Second, these findings may not be generalizable to horseback riders elsewhere in the United States because no comparable baseline information (e.g., hours of riding, hours of safety courses taken by decedents, and helmet use) is available.

Horseback riding requires coordination, timing, and communication of physical signals between horse and rider (5); alcohol use may impair equestrians, as it does operators of motor vehicles, by adversely effecting coordination and judgment and by lengthening reaction time (6). An alcohol-impaired rider may be unable to adjust to the horse's movements and may frighten the horse by unfamiliar actions. As with other transportation and recreational activities, use of helmets can prevent or reduce head injuries to persons riding horses (7,8), regardless of alcohol use. Horseback riders should wear a properly secured hard shell helmet lined with expanded polystyrene or similar material.

References
1. Bixby-Hammett DM. Accidents in equestrian sports. Am Fam Physician 1987;36:209–14.
2. Bixby-Hammett D, Brooks WH. Common injuries in horseback riding. Sports Med 1990;9:36–47.
3. Smith SM, Goodman RA, Thacker SB, Burton AH, Parsons JE, Hudson P. Alcohol and fatal injuries: temporal patterns. Am J Prev Med 1989;5:296–302.
4. Waller JA. Nonhighway injury fatalities—I. The roles of alcohol and problem drinking, drugs and medical impairment. J Chronic Dis 1972:25:33–45.
5. De Benedette V. People and horses: the risk of riding. Physician Sports Medicine 1989; 17:250–4.
6. Maull KI. Alcohol abuse: its implications in trauma care. South Med J 1982;75:794–8.
7. CDC. Injuries associated with horseback riding—United States, 1987 and 1988 MMWR 1990;39:329–32.
8. Grossman JA, Kulund DN, Miller CW, et al. Equestrian injuries: results of a prospective study. JAMA 1978;240:1881–2.

Tree Stand-Related Injuries Among Deer Hunters — Georgia, 1979–1989

Tree stand-related injuries can occur when a deer hunter unintentionally discharges a firearm while carrying it up to or down from a tree stand or upon impact after a fall. Hunters also can sustain fractures, sprains, strains, contusions, lacerations, internal injuries, and concussions when they fall from the tree stand, fall while descending or climbing the stand, or are injured when the stand collapses. In Georgia, such injuries accounted for 36% of all reported hunting injuries and for 20% of hunting-related fatalities. Hunter-safety courses in Georgia now require instruction on tree stand safety.

—MMWR Vol. 38/No. 41, October 20, 1989, pp. 697–700

Tree Stand-Related Injuries Among Deer Hunters —
Georgia, 1979–1989

Tree stands are elevated platforms used for hunting large game; they provide an expanded field of vision while minimizing ground scent. To characterize unintentional hunting injuries associated with the use of tree stands, the Georgia Department of Human Resources and the Georgia Department of Natural Resources (GDNR) studied all tree stand-related deer hunting injuries (reported on Georgia's mandatory Uniform Hunter Casualty Report form) for the 10 hunting seasons (mid-September through mid-January) during 1979–1989. A tree stand-related injury was defined as any injury associated with any device used to hunt deer from a tree. The number of big game (deer, bear, and turkey) hunting licenses issued in Georgia from the 1979–80 through the 1988–89 seasons was obtained from the Fishing and Game Licensing Bureau, GDNR.

During the 1979–1989 hunting seasons, 594 deer hunting-related injuries (including 85 fatal injuries) were reported in Georgia—a mean rate of 24.9 deer hunter injuries per 100,000 hunting licenses sold per year (range: 11.2–32.4) (Figure 1). Of these, 214 (36%) were tree stand-related (8.9 tree stand-related injuries per 100,000 hunting licenses sold per year [range: 2.4–13.7]) (Figure 1); 17 (8%) of these were fatal.

FIGURE 1. Tree stand-related injury rates per 100,000 licensed hunters — Georgia, 1979–1989

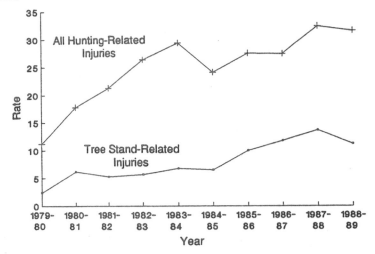

All the tree stand-related injuries occurred during hunting season. Tree stand-related injuries occurred in 89 (56%) of the 159 counties in Georgia; however, 24 (11%) injured hunters were residents of one of the five bordering states. The median age of injured hunters was 38 years (range: 8–72 years). Of nine who were <16 years of age, four were hunting without the supervision of an adult ≥21 years of age.

The type of hunting weapon was known for 178 tree stand-related injured hunters: 139 (78%) were hunting with a rifle; 23 (13%), with a bow and arrow; and 16 (9%), with a shotgun. Fractures and strains or sprains were the most commonly reported injuries (Table 1). Cervical spine fractures accounted for 16 (10%) of the fractures. Injuries to the trunk and extremities included fractures of the lumbar vertebrae, ribs, wrists, and ankles.

TABLE 1. Tree stand-related injuries among 214 deer hunters, by selected characteristics — Georgia, 1979–1989

Characteristic	No.	(%)	Characteristic	No.	(%)
Age (yrs)			**Type of injury***		
≤16	9	(4)	Fracture	156	(73)
17–35	114	(53)	Strain/sprain	21	(10)
36–64	84	(39)	Contusion	16	(7)
≥65	5	(2)	Laceration	13	(6)
Unknown	2	(1)	Internal[†]	13	(6)
Sex			Concussion	4	(2)
Male	198	(93)	Unknown	5	(2)
Female	16	(7)	**Location of injury***		
Type of tree stand			Trunk/back	112	(52)
Permanent	69	(32)	Lower extremity	78	(36)
Portable	48	(22)	Upper extremity	35	(16)
Unknown	97	(45)	Head and neck[§]	35	(16)
			Multiple sites	77	(36)

*Total may add to >100% because multiple sites are not exclusive of other sites.
[†]Includes pneumothorax and splenic laceration or rupture.
[§]Includes the cervical spine, face, and mouth.

Unintentional discharges of firearms caused 27 tree stand-related injuries and eight (47%) of the 17 fatalities. The firearm discharges occurred while the hunters were carrying their firearms up to or down from a tree stand or on impact after a fall.

One hundred eleven (52%) hunters were injured by falling from a tree stand, 49 (23%) fell while descending from a tree stand, and 40 (19%) fell while climbing to a tree stand; for 14 (7%), this information was unknown. Mechanical failure (i.e., collapse of the tree stand or its steps) occurred in 68 (32%) of the incidents. Eleven (5%) hunters reported they had fallen asleep in their tree stand immediately before falling, and eight (4%) either admitted to or were suspected of being intoxicated at the time of their incident.

For 65 injured hunters, information regarding participation in a hunter-safety course was indicated on the report form: 43 (66%) had not completed such a course. None of the 214 injured hunters were wearing a safety harness or seat-belt device at the time of injury.

Reported by: J Brown, Georgia Dept of Natural Resources; RK Sikes, DVM, State Epidemiologist, Georgia Dept of Human Resources. Div of Field Svcs, Epidemiology Program Office; Epidemiology Br, Div of Injury Epidemiology and Control, Center for Environmental Health and Injury Control, CDC.

Editorial Note: In previous reports on injuries among the approximately 20 million recreational hunters in North America, the role of tree stand-related injuries has not been emphasized (*1–5*). This investigation found that, in Georgia, tree stand-related injuries accounted for 36% of all reported hunting injuries and for 20% of hunting-related fatalities and that morbidity was substantial—73% of those injured sustained fractures (including fractures of the cervical or lumbar vertebrae).

In 1987, the North American Association of Hunter Safety Coordinators received reports of unintentional firearm injuries in 1792 hunters in 47 states and nine Canadian provinces—a rate of 9.2 firearm injuries per 100,000 licenses sold (*1*). Twenty-seven percent of injured hunters were <21 years of age, and 66% had not completed a hunter safety course. Younger hunters may be at higher risk for firearm injuries (*2–5*), suggesting that inexperience and poor judgment contribute to injuries. In most states, a hunter-safety course is required before a hunting license is issued. In Georgia, a mandatory hunting training law (enacted in 1977) requires only persons who were born after 1960 and are ≥16 years old to successfully complete the approved hunter-education course to obtain a hunting license; persons who were born before 1961 or who are <16 years old are exempted from the course (*6*).

Although safety devices (e.g., belts and harnesses) could prevent injuries from falls in Georgia, none of the tree stand-related injured hunters were wearing safety devices. In addition, some injuries resulting from mechanical failure of tree stands might have been prevented if hunters had inspected construction (including nails and bolts) and pretested the tree stands before use. The injuries and fatalities resulting from the unintentional discharge of weapons might have been prevented if the hunters had unloaded the guns or bows during placement and had used pull-up cords to raise or lower the weapons.

Hunter-safety courses in Georgia now require instruction on tree stand safety, with an emphasis on use of safety devices and pull-up cords to move unloaded weapons. Pamphlets (*7*) and a videocassette (*8*) that promote tree stand safety are commercially available.*

References
1. North American Association of Hunter Safety Coordinators. Hunting accident report, with graphics of 1983–1987 data. Seattle: Outdoor Empire Publishing, 1987.
2. Carter GL. Accidental firearm fatalities and injuries among recreational hunters. Ann Emerg Med 1989;18:406–9.
3. Cole TB, Patetta MJ. Hunting firearm injuries, North Carolina. Am J Public Health 1988; 78:1585–6.
4. Morgan PL, Hudson P. Accidental firearm injuries in North Carolina, 1976–80. Am J Public Health 1986;76:1120–3.
5. Ornechult L, Eriksson A. Accidental firearm fatalities during hunting. Am J Forensic Med Pathol 1987;8:112–9.
6. Georgia Department of Natural Resources, Game and Fish Division, Law Enforcement Section. Georgia hunter evaluation handbook. Seattle: Outdoor Empire Publishing, 1987:2.
7. Richter F. Tree stand guide. Murray, Kentucky: National Bowhunter Education Foundation, 1988.
8. Poland TM. Tree stands: above all safety first [Videocassette]. Columbia, South Carolina: Pebblecreek Production, 1987.

---

*Mention of these products is for reader information only and does not imply endorsement by the Public Health Service or the U.S. Department of Health and Human Services.

Serious Eye Injuries Associated with Fireworks — United States, 1990–1994

Fireworks—especially bottle rockets—continue to cause serious eye injuries each year. The Centers for Disease Control and Prevention supports the United States Eye Injury Registry's recommendation that people should attend professionally conducted public displays of fireworks or should 1) never use bottle rockets, 2) make sure that fireworks operators, bystanders, and spectators wear eye protection, 3) never allow young children to use fireworks, 4) supervise older children when using fireworks, 5) use fireworks only outdoors, 6) always keep water nearby to douse fires and malfunctioning fireworks, 7) read and follow carefully fireworks instructions, and 8) not relight malfunctioning fireworks.

—MMWR Vol. 44/No. 24, June 23, 1995, pp. 449–52

Serious Eye Injuries Associated with Fireworks —
United States, 1990–1994

Eye injuries caused by fireworks are often severe and can cause permanently reduced visual acuity or blindness. Findings from the National Electronic Injury Surveillance System database maintained by the U.S. Consumer Product Safety Commission (CPSC) indicate that approximately 12,000 persons are treated each year in U.S. emergency departments because of fireworks-related injuries; of these, an estimated 20% are eye injuries. To improve characterization of fireworks-related eye injuries, data were analyzed from the United States Eye Injury Registry (USEIR) for July 1990–December 1994 and from the Eye Injury Registry of Alabama (EIRA) for August 1982–July 1989. This report summarizes the findings of these analyses.

United States Eye Injury Registry

USEIR, a nonprofit organization sponsored by the Helen Keller Eye Research Foundation, is a federation of state eye registries that uses a standardized form to obtain voluntarily reported data on eye injuries and to obtain 6-month follow-up information. Reports are made by ophthalmologists to the USEIR database in Birmingham, Alabama. The primary purpose of USEIR is to provide prospective, population-based, epidemiologic data to improve the prevention and control of eye injuries. The registry contains information only for patients who have sustained a serious eye injury, defined as "an injury resulting in permanent and significant, structural or functional ocular change." USEIR comprises 39 state registry affiliates (representing 89% of the U.S. population); 32 states registered injuries during 1990–1994, and 27 states reported fireworks-related injuries during this period.

From July 1990 through December 1994, a total of 4575 serious eye injuries from all causes were reported to USEIR; of the 274 (6%) fireworks-related injuries, 255 (93%) were unintentional injuries. Persons injured by fireworks were aged 4–63 years (median: 15 years); 211 (77%) were males. The largest proportion (123 [45%]) of injured persons were bystanders; 96 (35%) were fireworks operators, and for 55 (20%), status was unknown. Most (219 [80%]) injuries occurred during the Independence Day holiday period*; 44 (16%) occurred during the New Year's holiday period*, and 11 (4%) at other times. Most (67%) injuries occurred at home; injuries also occurred in recreational settings (14%), on a street or highway (5%), and in parking lots or occupational settings (1%). Location was unknown for 13%.

Most injuries were caused by bottle rockets (58%) (Figure 1). Bottle rockets accounted for 68% of the injuries to bystanders.

Eye Injury Registry of Alabama

A retrospective review was begun in 1989 of severely injured persons registered from August 1982 through July 1989 through the EIRA, the first state registry of USEIR. Reports to the EIRA are made by Alabama ophthalmologists. Data were obtained from EIRA standard report forms and from direct interviews with each injured person and/or family members.

Of the 70 fireworks-related injuries reported, 40 (57%) occurred during the Independence Day holiday period, and 27 (39%) occurred during the New Year's holiday period. These injuries resulted in legal blindness in 31 (44%) injured persons; in addition, enucleation was required for seven (10%). Bottle rockets accounted for 58 (83%) injuries, including eight of 10 injuries resulting in permanent damage to the optic nerve and all those resulting in enucleation.

---

*The number of days for the holiday period varied each year.

FIGURE 1. Percentage of fireworks-related serious eye injuries, by type of firework — United States Eye Injury Registry, 1990–1994

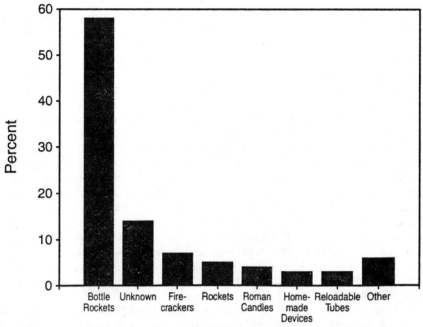

Type of Firework

Patients who sustained eye injuries resulting from bottle rockets reported that factors associated with their injuries included product misuse, (e.g., the intentional aiming of the device at others ["bottle rocket wars"] and throwing the device after it had been lit but before ignition), device malfunction (especially immediate explosion after ignition), erratic flight characteristics even when used according to manufacturers' instructions, and device ricochet off hard surfaces (e.g., a car or the street).

Reported by: S Brown, MPH, CD Witherspoon, MD, R Morris, MD, SM Hamilton, MD, FI Camesasca, MD, JA Kimble, MD, United States Eye Injury Registry, Birmingham, Alabama. Directorate for Epidemiology and Health Sciences, Div of Hazard Analysis, US Consumer Product Safety Commission. Div of Unintentional Injury Prevention, National Center for Injury Prevention and Control, CDC.

Editorial Note: Irreversible consequences—including reduced visual acuity and blindness—can result from the use of consumer fireworks, especially bottle rockets. Analysis of the USEIR database indicated that a high proportion of fireworks-related injuries occurred among young males—a finding consistent with previous reports (*1,2*). These findings are similar to the results of a study in Washington in which injuries were associated with improper use (both intentional and unintentional); product malfunctions (e.g., short fuses, erratic flight, or tip-over), and high temperature (*2*).

Consumer fireworks—including bottle rockets (classified as 1.4G [formally known as Class C] fireworks)—have been banned in 10 states (Arizona, Connecticut, Delaware, Georgia, Massachusetts, Minnesota, New Jersey, New York, Rhode Island, and

Vermont). Six states (Illinois, Iowa, Maine, Maryland, Ohio, and Pennsylvania) permit the use only of sparklers and other novelties (e.g., poppers, wheels, and snaps). The District of Columbia and 32 states allow at least some 1.4G fireworks to be sold. Nevada and Hawaii have no laws regulating fireworks except for local ordinances. The CPSC has banned firecrackers with >50 mg pyrotechnic composition (including cherry bombs, M-80s, and silver salutes) designed to detonate on or near the ground and reloadable shell devices with diameters exceeding 1.75 inches; bottle-rockets can contain up to 130 mg pyrotechnic composition.

Because of the risks for injury associated with bottle rockets and other fireworks, several organizations have made specific recommendations regarding their use. USEIR recommends that persons attend public fireworks displays; however, if persons choose to use fireworks, USEIR recommends that they not use bottle rockets, and when other fireworks are used, eye protection should be worn by operators, bystanders, and spectators. CPSC and USEIR also advise that young children should never use fireworks, older children should be supervised when using fireworks, fireworks should be used only outdoors, a source of water should always be nearby for fire and to douse malfunctioning fireworks, instructions should be read and followed carefully, and malfunctioning fireworks should not be relit.

Several states have prohibited bottle rocket sales, and such bans are supported by the American Academy of Ophthalmology (3), American Academy of Pediatrics (4), and American Public Health Association (5). Despite the advisories regarding the dangers of fireworks use and state bans on use, fireworks continue to cause serious eye injuries—fireworks purchasers often cross state borders during holiday seasons to obtain fireworks that are illegal in their own states. In addition, because USEIR is a voluntary registry and not all states are affiliated, the numbers presented in this report may underestimate the problem nationally. CDC, concurring with the USEIR recommendations, suggests that health-care providers urge patients and their families to attend professionally conducted public displays of fireworks.

References

1. CDC. Fireworks-related injuries—Marion County, Indiana, 1986–1991. MMWR 1992;41:451–4.
2. CDC. Fireworks-related injuries—Washington. MMWR 1983;32:285–6.
3. Eye Safety and Sports Ophthalmology Committee. Fireworks remain serious health hazard and cause of blindness. San Francisco: American Academy of Ophthalmology, May 1995.
4. Committee on Injury and Poison Prevention. Children and fireworks. Pediatr 1991;88:652–3.
5. American Public Health Association. Resolution 9111—banning bottle rockets: prevention of ocular injuries. In: American Public Health Association. Public policy statements of the American Public Health Association. Washington, DC: American Public Health Association, 1994: 482–3.

Fireworks-Related Injuries — Marion County, Indiana, 1986–1991

During the 6-year study period, 159 persons were injured by fireworks in Marion County, with nearly half of the injuries occurring among children and adolescents 14 years of age and younger. No fireworks should be considered completely safe for children. Educational efforts need to be directed toward the parents of young children.

—MMWR Vol. 41/No. 25, June 26, 1992, pp. 451–4

Fireworks-Related Injuries —
Marion County, Indiana, 1986–1991

Based on data from the Consumer Product Safety Commission's (CPSC) National Electronic Injury Surveillance System, fireworks-related injuries accounted for an estimated 12,400 emergency room visits during 1990 in the United States (1); two thirds of fireworks-related injuries occur during the 4-week period surrounding Independence Day. Since 1986, to better characterize fireworks-related injuries and to improve local health education and prevention efforts, the Marion County (Indiana) Health Department (MCHD) has conducted surveillance of fireworks-related injuries. This report summarizes surveillance results for 1986–1991.

Marion County (1990 population: 797,159) includes metropolitan Indianapolis. Each year, the MCHD collects data on demographic characteristics of injured persons, nature of the injury, type of device, and circumstances surrounding the incident (e.g., adult presence at time of injury) from all eight area hospital emergency rooms from June 27 through July 11.

During the 6-year period, 159 persons were reportedly injured by fireworks in Marion County. Fewest injuries (16) occurred during 1988; injuries peaked (37) during 1990. Most injuries (76 [48%]) occurred among children and adolescents aged <15 years; 32 (20%) occurred among adolescents and young adults aged 15–24 years, and 45 (28%), among adults aged 25–44 years. Males accounted for 74% of the injuries.

Burns were the most common (127 [72%] of 177) type of fireworks-related injury reported; 11% of injuries were lacerations, 9%, abrasions, 2%, puncture wounds, and 6%, other injuries. By site of injury, hands/fingers were most commonly involved (61 [34%] of 177) followed by eyes (17%) and the face (12%); however, during 1988, eyes (seven [44%] of 16) were the most frequently reported site of injury.

Fireworks devices most often associated with injuries varied by age group. Among children <5 years of age, sparklers were the leading cause of injury (54%), followed by firecrackers (23%), bottle rockets (11%), twisters or "jumping jacks" (8%), and other devices (4%). Of all sparkler-related injuries, 42% occurred among children aged <5 years. For children aged 5–14 years, firecrackers (34%) ranked first, followed by twisters (18%), sparklers (16%), bottle rockets (14%), and other devices (18%); most injuries involving twisters (53%) occurred among persons in this age group. For young adults aged 15–24 years, bottle rockets (35%) and firecrackers (16%) combined caused more than half of the injuries. Adults aged 25–44 years were injured most frequently by bottle rockets (33%), firecrackers (28%), and sparklers (23%). Of the five persons aged ≥45 years, three were injured by firecrackers.

The most frequent injury-causing event reported involving other fireworks-related devices was lighting gunpowder, which accounted for injuries to eight persons aged 15–24 years. During the 6-year period, 53% of minors injured by fireworks were under adult supervision at the time of the injury.

Reported by: DS Joseph, MS, Marion County Health Dept; ML Fleissner, DrPH, State Epidemiologist, Indiana State Board of Health. Unintentional Injuries Section, Epidemiology Br, Div of Injury Control, National Center for Environmental Health and Injury Control, CDC.

Editorial Note: Although use of commercial fireworks rarely results in injuries, the private use of fireworks during the Independence Day holiday period has been associated with an increasing trend of substantial injuries. The National Fire Protection Association (NFPA) used CPSC data to estimate that, in the United States, the average annual number of emergency room visits resulting from fireworks use increased at least 48% during 1986–1990, compared with 1974–1978 (1). The NFPA also characterized the substantial economic and public health impact resulting from fireworks: during 1988, fireworks accounted for an estimated 44,500 fires that resulted in 20 deaths and $41 million in direct property damage.

The demographic characteristics of persons most frequently injured by fireworks in Marion County are consistent with national findings and with previous studies from Washington state (2–4). Young males were most frequently injured; however, for fireworks — as well as for most other injury causes — it is not possible to determine whether young males are at increased risk for injury or whether their injury patterns reflect increased exposure to injury-causing events.

In Marion County, injuries were associated with every category of fireworks. The relation of age of person injured to type of fireworks device was also consistent with national findings. For example, sparkler injuries were a substantial problem for young children (2); adults were more likely to be injured by aerial devices such as bottle rockets. A previous report from Washington indicated that, among all age groups, fireworks-related injuries were associated with firecrackers and aerial devices and with a variety of misuse behaviors (e.g., relighting, throwing, holding in hand, and bending over to light). For children aged <16 years, lack of adult supervision was a significant risk factor for injury (odds ratio = 11.5; 95% confidence interval = 2.8–100.6) (3).

Current federal, state, and local laws regulating sales of fireworks to private persons are inconsistent and, therefore, undermine enforcement. For example, fireworks can be transported easily from legal to illegal jurisdictions. Increased availability of fireworks, legally or illegally, can increase related injuries. For example, during 1982, Washington standardized restrictions on fireworks sales to provide uniform availability of firecrackers and aerial devices statewide (5). Before the law change, explosive ground devices, aerial devices, and exploding firecrackers containing less than 50 mg of gunpowder were available only on American Indian reservations; the new law made these devices available outside reservations as well. As a consequence following the change in law, surveillance conducted by the Washington Department of Health documented a significant increase in the number of fireworks-related injuries reported by 15 hospitals in nine counties (from 39 in 1981 to 88 in 1982; $p < 0.001$) (5).

Both legal and illegal fireworks are associated with injuries. During 1989, 73% of fireworks-related injuries reported through the CPSC system were associated with devices legally acquired under federal law (2). However, illegal fireworks may cause more severe injuries; during 1989, two thirds of injuries requiring hospitalization were associated with fireworks illegal under federal law (2).

In addition to stronger and more uniform restrictions on the availability of certain fireworks, educational efforts should also be employed to reduce injuries. For example, during the 1988 Independence Day holiday period, Marion County had the fewest number of fireworks-related injuries for 1986–1991; at the same time, however, a severe drought in Indiana prompted local public safety officials to discourage fireworks use — a message that was well publicized by the local media.

No fireworks should be considered completely safe for children. Educational efforts directed toward parents of young children have been effective in support of other injury-prevention campaigns such as the use of child safety seats. The American Academy of Pediatrics' Committee on Injury Prevention and Control recommends similar efforts to reduce injuries associated with sparklers and other fireworks that have special appeal to children (6). The CPSC has developed guidelines for parents living in areas that allow the sale of fireworks for personal use (see box) (4).

The MCHD provides its surveillance data to local media and interest groups (e.g., state and local fire marshals and state legislators) concerned with fireworks safety. In addition, all Marion County hospitals receive an overall report on the incidence of fireworks-related injuries and associated health-care concerns.

Recommendations to Parents Regarding Personal Fireworks Safety

- Do not allow younger children to play with fireworks under any circumstances. Remember that fireworks are not toys for children. The sparkler, considered by many as the ideal "safe" fireworks for the young, burns at very high temperatures and can easily ignite clothing. Children cannot appreciate the danger involved and cannot act correctly in the case of emergency.

- Closely supervise older children who are permitted to use fireworks. Do not allow any running or boisterous play while fireworks are being used.

- Before using any fireworks, read and follow all warning instructions printed on the label.

- Light fireworks outdoors in a clear area away from houses and flammable materials (e.g., gasoline cans).

- Keep a bucket of water nearby for emergencies and for dousing fireworks that do not go off.

- Do not try to relight or handle malfunctioning fireworks. Soak them with water and throw them away.

- Be sure other people are out of range before lighting fireworks.

- Never ignite fireworks in a container, especially a glass or metal container.

- Store fireworks in a dry, cool place. Check instructions for special storage directions.

Source: Consumer Product Safety Commission.

References
1. National Fire Protection Association. NFPA: fire facts. Quincy, Massachusetts: National Fire Protection Association, April 1991.
2. National Fire Protection Association. NFPA: fire facts. Quincy, Massachusetts: National Fire Protection Association, April 1990.
3. McFarland LV, Harris JR, Kobayashi JM, Dicker RC. Risk factors for fireworks-related injury in Washington state. JAMA 1984;251:3251–4.
4. Berger LR, Kalishman S, Rivara FP. Injuries from fireworks. Pediatrics 1985;75:877–82.
5. CDC. Fireworks-related injuries—Washington. MMWR 1983;32:285–6.
6. Committee on Injury Prevention and Control, American Academy of Pediatrics. Children and fireworks. Pediatrics 1991;88:652–3.

Playground-Related Injuries in Preschool-Aged Children — United States, 1983–1987

Playground safety improvements are needed to reduce childhood injuries, particularly falls, which account for 60% of playground equipment-related injuries. Injury control interventions include 1) installing playground equipment over appropriate surfaces, 2) locating the equipment away from obstructions and covering protrusions, 3) properly anchoring the equipment and checking its integrity, 4) instructing and supervising children, 5) limiting the height of playground equipment, and 6) urging parents to consider the safety aspects of playgrounds in day care centers, schools, and public areas before allowing their children to use them.

—MMWR Vol. 37/No. 41, October 21, 1988, pp. 629–32

Playground-Related Injuries
in Preschool-Aged Children — United States, 1983–1987

From 1983 to 1987, nearly 6.72 million emergency room visits in the United States were for product-related injuries among preschool children 1–4 years old.* Approximately 305,000 (4.5%) of these injuries involved playground equipment. These playground equipment-related injuries occurred most frequently at home (38.3%), in sports or recreation settings (29.4%), or at school (8.9%) (Table 1). Of the 82,108 injuries in preschool-aged children attending day care (coded as occurring at school), 27,232 (33.2%) were related to playground equipment (Table 1).

TABLE 1. Playground-related and other injuries in preschool-aged children, by locale — United States, 1983–1987

Locale	Playground-related injuries		Other injuries	
	No.	(%)	No.	(%)
Any home*	116,963	(38.3)	5,262,909	(82.1)
Sports or recreation setting	89,631	(29.4)	74,269	(1.2)
School	27,232	(8.9)	54,876	(0.9)
Other[†]	24,383	(8.0)	350,972	(5.5)
Unknown	47,072	(15.4)	668,570	(10.4)
Total	305,281	(100.0)	6,411,596	(100.0)

*Includes injuries occurring inside or outside a house, farmhouse (not farm-related), apartment, condominium, or mobile home.
[†]Includes injuries occurring at a street, highway, store, office building, restaurant, church, farm, or industrial place.

Most preschool-aged children with injuries involving school playground equipment were 3 or 4 years old and male (Table 2). A higher proportion of playground-related injuries occurred in the spring than at other times of the year (Table 2). Forty percent of playground-related injuries were associated with climbing apparatus, and two thirds of injuries were to the head and neck (Table 2).

Lacerations (38.5%), contusions or abrasions (26.8%), fractures (16.8%), strains or sprains (4.4%), and concussions (1.7%) were most commonly reported (Table 2). Head and neck injuries were primarily lacerations (55.7%) and contusions or abrasions (23.7%). Injury to the extremities and trunk included mostly fractures, contusions or abrasions, and strains or sprains (upper extremity—62.4%, 22.2%, and 12.2%; lower extremity—31.4%, 42.2%, and 15.4%; trunk—27.7%, 51.2%, and 9.2%, respectively). Approximately 5.3% of preschool-aged children treated in emergency rooms for playground-related injuries required hospitalization.

---

*This estimate is based on data from the National Electronic Injury Surveillance System (NEISS) of the U.S. Consumer Product Safety Commission (CPSC). Sixty-two hospitals with emergency rooms located throughout the United States contribute to this data base. When weighted, the reports from NEISS reflect national estimates of persons with product-related injuries treated in hospital emergency rooms.

TABLE 2. School playground-related injuries in children aged 1–4 years, by selected items — United States, 1983–1987

Characteristic	Playground-related injuries		Characteristic	Playground-related injuries	
	No.*	(%)		No.*	(%)
Age (yrs)			Location of injury		
1	1,154	(4.2)	Head and neck[§]	18,099	(66.5)
2	4,557	(16.7)	Upper extremity	5,021	(18.4)
3	9,015	(33.1)	Lower extremity	2,027	(7.4)
4	12,506	(45.9)	Trunk	1,858	(6.8)
Sex			Multiple sites	228	(0.8)
Male	15,195	(55.8)			
Female	12,038	(44.2)	Injury diagnosis		
Season			Laceration	10,471	(38.5)
Spring	9,211	(33.8)	Contusion/abrasion	7,309	(26.8)
Summer	5,279	(19.4)	Fracture	4,581	(16.8)
Fall	6,275	(23.0)	Strain/sprain	1,209	(4.4)
Winter	6,466	(23.7)	Concussion	468	(1.7)
Type of equipment			Other	3,081	(11.3)
Climbing apparatus	11,027	(40.5)	Unknown	114	(0.4)
Slide/sliding board[†]	7,043	(25.9)			
Swing/swing set	4,956	(18.2)			
Seesaw/teeterboard	1,302	(4.8)			
Other	2,905	(10.7)			

*These are national estimates of product-related injuries treated in hospital emergency rooms using data from the National Electronic Injury Surveillance System.
[†]Excluding swimming pools and ground water slides.
[§]Including the face and mouth.

Reported by: Div of Injury Epidemiology and Control, Center for Environmental Health and Injury Control, CDC.

Editorial Note: By 1984, more than 11 million children attended day-care facilities (1). The potential injury hazards of organized day care and day-care playgrounds have been documented (2–5). The NEISS data suggest that further improvements in playground safety are needed to reduce playground-related injuries.

NEISS provides a data base for estimating injuries associated with playground equipment in young children in day-care facilities. However, these data are limited in that, by using "school" as the location to represent day-care playgrounds, they exclude children injured in day care at a home, church, or building other than a school. Conversely, some injuries that reportedly took place at school possibly occurred to children using a school playground but not attending day care. Interpreting these data is also difficult because the type, size, and cost of equipment at a school playground differ from those used in homes, churches, or private day care. Thus, the distribution by type of equipment in the overall day-care environment may vary considerably from that described here.

A CPSC-sponsored hazard analysis showed that falls to the ground surface account for 60% of playground equipment-related injuries (*6*). A 1-foot fall directly on the head onto concrete or asphalt or a 4-foot fall onto packed earth can be fatal (*7–9*). In contrast, surfaces made of energy-absorbing mats or loose materials such as wood chips or sand may reduce the likelihood of head injury even from falls of 8 feet (*7,8*). Yet over 48% of day-care playground equipment is not installed over impact-absorbing surfaces (*2,3*). Although in some cases the Occupational Safety and Health Administration requires that guard rails be installed to protect workers as low as 4 feet above ground level, no such protective legislation exists for children on playground equipment, some of which is more than 10 feet above the ground (*8*).

Injury control programs should address the safety aspects of public and other playgrounds for all ages. According to NEISS data, 994,678 injuries in all age groups from 1983 to 1987 were associated with playground equipment; 243,807 (24.5%) of these injuries occurred at schools, and 257,070 (25.8%), at places of recreation. Recommendations to improve playground safety include installing playground equipment over energy-absorbing surfaces, locating the equipment away from obstructions, properly anchoring the equipment, checking the integrity of the equipment frequently, covering protrusions, removing broken equipment promptly, and instructing and supervising children in proper playground use (*10,11*). If wood chips or sand are used as surfacing, they should be well maintained and not allowed to compact or fall below an adequate depth. Limiting the height of playground equipment may also be helpful. Parents should consider the safety aspects of playgrounds in day-care centers, schools, and public areas before allowing their children to use them.

References
 1. The Child Day Care Infectious Disease Study Group. Public health considerations of infectious diseases in child day care centers. J Pediatr 1984;105:683–701.
 2. O'Connor MA, Boyle WE Jr, O'Connor GT, Letellier R. Injury prevention practices in daycare centers. Presented at the 115th annual meeting of the American Public Health Association, New Orleans, Louisiana, October 18–22, 1987.
 3. Davis WS, McCarthy PL. Safety in day-care centers [Abstract]. Am J Dis Child 1988;142:386.
 4. Aronson SS. Injuries in child care. Young Child 1983;38:19–20.
 5. Landman PF, Landman GB. Accidental injuries in children in day-care centers. Am J Dis Child 1987;141:292–3.
 6. Rutherford GW Jr. Injuries associated with public playground equipment. Washington, DC: US Consumer Product Safety Commission, 1978.
 7. Mahajan BM, Beine WB. Impact attenuation performance of surfaces installed under playground equipment: report to the Consumer Product Safety Commission. Washington, DC: US Department of Commerce, National Bureau of Standards, Feb. 1979; publication no. NBSIR 79-1707.
 8. Reichelderfer TE, Overbach A, Greensher J. Unsafe playgrounds [Letter]. Pediatrics 1979;64:962–3.
 9. Sweeney TB. X-rated playgrounds? [Letter]. Pediatrics 1979;64:961.
10. US Consumer Product Safety Commission. A handbook for public playground safety: general guidelines for new and existing playgrounds. Vol I. Washington, DC: US Consumer Product Safety Commission, 1986.
11. US Consumer Product Safety Commission. Play happy, play safely: playground equipment guide for teachers, park and recreation directors, parents, youth leaders, and other concerned adults. Washington, DC: US Consumer Product Safety Commission, 1979.

Poisonings

Unintentional Poisoning Mortality — United States, 1980–1986

Unintentional poisoning mortality is predominantly a problem among young adults, particularly men 20–39 years of age. Through its Drug Abuse Warning Network (DAWN), the National Institute on Drug Abuse monitors emergency departments and medical examiner's offices in selected locations for drug-related emergency visits and deaths. According to DAWN data for 1987, cocaine was the most frequently reported drug involved in emergency visits, and heroin/morphine and cocaine each were involved in more than one-third of deaths. Persons aged 20–39 years accounted for 70% of all drug-abuse emergency visits and 65% of all drug-abuse deaths.

—MMWR Vol. 38/No. 10, March 17, 1989, pp. 153–7

Unintentional Poisoning Mortality — United States, 1980–1986

March 19–25, 1989, marks the 28th annual observance of National Poison Prevention Week (NPPW). NPPW is intended to alert the public to the problem of unintentional poisoning (the ingestion, injection, inhalation, or absorption of a chemical agent that results in unanticipated illness or death), the fifth leading cause of unintentional injury deaths in the United States. The traditional goal of NPPW is prevention of poisoning among children. Although childhood poisoning mortality has decreased in recent years, morbidity associated with poisoning in this age group remains a major public health problem. In 1987, 731,954 poisoning exposures among children <6 years of age were reported to the American Association of Poison Control Centers' National Data Collection System; 22 of these children died, and 107,844 others became ill (1). The number of exposures to household medicines and chemicals can be reduced by more widespread use of safety-packaged products by parents and other caretakers of children. The following report focuses on unintentional poisoning mortality among young adults, including poisonings from both the medical and nonmedical use of drugs.

Unintentional poisoning deaths in the United States were analyzed for 1980–1986 using final mortality data from CDC's National Center for Health Statistics (NCHS).* Age-adjusted mortality rates were directly standardized to the 1980 U.S. population.

From 1980 through 1986, the mortality rate of unintentional poisonings in the United States increased from 1.9 to 2.3 deaths/100,000 population (Figure 1). This

FIGURE 1. Rate of death from unintentional poisonings* per 100,000 persons — United States, 1980–1986

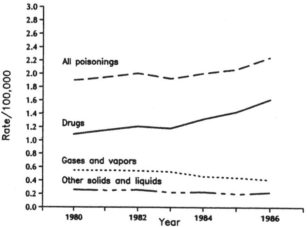

*ICD-9 codes: drugs (E850–E858), other solids and liquids (E860–E866), gases and vapors (E867–E869).

---

*NCHS codes the underlying cause of death according to the International Classification of Diseases (ICD). The ICD Ninth Revision (ICD-9) has been in use since the beginning of 1979. NCHS uses the ICD-9 codes E850–E858 for unintentional drug poisoning deaths, such as overdoses, regardless of whether the drug was administered for medical reasons. NCHS codes other drug-related deaths as deaths due to drug dependence (ICD-9 code 304), nondependent drug abuse (305.2–305.9), suicide by drugs (E950.0–E950.5), and poisoning by drugs in which the intentions of the decedent are undetermined (E980.0–E980.5).

7-year trend appears to be explained by a 49% increase in the rate of deaths from drug poisoning, including drugs used for both medical and nonmedical purposes. Mortality rates of unintentional poisoning by other solids and liquids and by gases and vapors decreased by 15% and 25%, respectively, during 1980–1986. In 1986, the most recent year for which NCHS mortality data are available, drug poisonings accounted for 1.6 deaths/100,000 persons and 73% of all unintentional poisoning deaths (Table 1).

In 1986, the leading causes of fatal unintentional drug poisonings were opiates and related narcotics and local anesthetics including cocaine (Table 2). Most of the fatal poisonings by other solids and liquids were due to alcohol ingestion (352 deaths). Exposure to motor vehicle exhaust (475 deaths) accounted for nearly half the deaths due to unintentional poisoning by gases and vapors.

TABLE 1. Number of deaths associated with unintentional poisonings, by type of poisoning* and year — United States, 1980–1986

| Year | Type of unintentional poisoning | | | Total |
	Drugs	Other solids & liquids	Gases & vapors	
1980	2492	597	1242	4331
1981	2668	575	1280	4523
1982	2862	612	1259	4733
1983	2866	516	1251	4633
1984	3266	542	1103	4911
1985	3612	479	1079	5170
1986	4187	544	1009	5740

*ICD-9 codes corresponding to type of unintentional poisoning: drugs (E850–E858), other solids and liquids (E860–E866), gases and vapors (E867–E869).

TABLE 2. Number of deaths from unintentional drug poisonings, by type of drug — United States, 1986

Type of drug	Deaths	ICD-9 code(s)
Opiates and related narcotics	930	E850.0
Local anesthetics including cocaine	624	E855.2
Nonnarcotic analgesics	349	E850.1–E850.9
Cardiovascular drugs	263	E858.3
Other psychotropic drugs	222	E851–E853, E854.1–E854.3
Antidepressants	154	E854.0
Antibiotics and other anti-infectives	69	E856, E857
Other drugs acting on the central and autonomic nervous systems	61	E855.0–E855.1, E855.3–E855.9
Other specified drugs	822	E858.0–E858.2, E858.4–E858.8
Unspecified drugs	693	E858.9
All	4187	E850–E858

The mortality rate of unintentional poisonings for males remained more than twice that for females during 1980–1986 (Table 3). The rates for blacks of both sexes were consistently higher than those for whites. In 1986, the rate for black males was 5.4 deaths/100,000 persons, and for white males, 3.2 deaths/100,000 persons.

TABLE 3. Unintentional poisoning deaths* and mortality rates per 100,000 population, by decedents' sex and age — United States, 1980–1986

Sex & age group (yrs)	1980		1982		1984		1986	
	No.	Rate	No.	Rate	No.	Rate	No.	Rate
Male								
0–4	63	0.8	57	0.6	60	0.7	51	0.6
5–9	13	0.2	10	0.1	10	0.1	14	0.2
10–19	217	1.1	161	0.8	145	0.8	175	1.0
20–29	930	4.5	1052	5.0	1002	4.7	1077	5.1
30–39	609	3.9	846	5.0	1074	5.9	1448	7.4
40–49	346	3.1	363	3.2	382	3.1	535	4.2
50–59	305	2.8	288	2.6	290	2.7	287	2.7
≥60	404	2.7	447	2.8	456	2.8	513	3.0
Total[†]	**2890**	**2.6**	**3224**	**2.9**	**3419**	**3.0**	**4105**	**3.5**
Age-adjusted[§]		2.7		2.8		2.9		3.3
Female								
0–4	42	0.5	47	0.6	38	0.4	42	0.5
5–9	10	0.1	11	0.1	12	0.2	10	0.1
10–19	105	0.5	82	0.4	73	0.4	74	0.4
20–29	292	1.4	292	1.4	318	1.5	304	1.4
30–39	219	1.4	254	1.5	290	1.6	380	1.9
40–49	171	1.5	205	1.7	183	1.4	207	1.5
50–59	205	1.7	206	1.7	181	1.5	153	1.3
≥60	397	1.9	410	1.9	395	1.8	464	2.0
Total[†]	**1441**	**1.2**	**1507**	**1.3**	**1490**	**1.2**	**1635**	**1.3**
Age-adjusted[§]		1.2		1.2		1.2		1.2

*ICD-9 codes corresponding to unintentional poisonings are E850–E869.
[†]Includes decedents with unknown ages.
[§]Standardized to the 1980 U.S. census population.

The highest mortality rates of unintentional poisonings for both blacks and whites were for young adult men (20–39 years of age). Men in this age group accounted for 40% of all unintentional poisoning deaths and 46% of all unintentional drug poisoning deaths during 1980–1986. In 1986, among young adult men, unintentional drug poisonings were responsible for 2065 deaths or 5.1 deaths/100,000 persons, an 85% increase from 1980.

In 1986, the leading causes of fatal unintentional drug poisonings for young adult men were opiates and related narcotics (619 deaths) and local anesthetics including cocaine (436 deaths). By comparison, in 1980, among young adult men, 213 deaths resulted from poisoning by opiates and related narcotics, and 73 deaths, from poisoning by local anesthetics including cocaine. In 1980 and 1986, additional deaths occurred among young adult men from unintentional poisonings by drug combinations, and an unknown number of these deaths involved opiates or cocaine.[†]

The mortality rate for unintentional poisonings among children <15 years of age was 0.3 deaths/100,000 persons in 1986, a 10% decrease from 1980. In 1986, 147 such deaths occurred among children <15 years of age, including 62 deaths from gases and vapors and 54 from drugs.

Reported by: Biometrics Br and Program Development and Implementation Br, Div of Injury Epidemiology and Control, Center for Environmental Health and Injury Control, CDC.

Editorial Note: Unintentional poisoning mortality is predominantly a problem of young adults, particularly men 20–39 years of age. NCHS data indicate that the misuse of drugs, primarily opiates and related narcotics and cocaine, was responsible for a substantial increase in such deaths among men in this age group from 1980 through 1986. The impact of drug use on mortality is only partially conveyed by enumeration of unintentional poisoning deaths (*2*). The mortality rate for young adult men rose during 1980–1986 for deaths attributed to drug dependence, nondependent drug abuse, and poisoning by drugs in which the intentions of the decedent are undetermined. For suicide by drugs, the mortality rate in young adult men remained nearly constant (1.6 deaths/100,000 persons in 1986) (NCHS, unpublished data).

The National Institute on Drug Abuse (NIDA) has reported increases in morbidity and mortality associated with nonmedical use of both heroin/morphine and cocaine during 1985–1987 (*3*). Through its Drug Abuse Warning Network (DAWN), NIDA monitors emergency departments and medical examiners' offices in selected locations for drug-related emergency visits and deaths. In 1987, cocaine was the most frequently reported drug involved in emergency visits, and heroin/morphine and cocaine each were involved in more than one third of deaths reported to DAWN. According to DAWN data for 1987, persons 20–39 years of age accounted for 70% of all drug-abuse emergency visits and 65% of all drug-abuse deaths (*4*).

Reducing unintentional poisoning mortality among young adults requires prevention programs and treatment efforts that focus on the use of illicit drugs. Although medical complications of illicit drug use often emerge early in adulthood, initiation of drug use during adolescence is an important risk factor for later hazardous use. This suggests that deterring or even delaying initiation of drug use among adolescents is an appropriate goal of prevention (*5*). However, the recent increase in unintentional drug poisoning deaths among young adults underscores the need for drug education and treatment that focus on illicit drug users who are 20–39 years of age.

References
1. Litovitz TL, Schmitz BF, Matyunas N, Martin TG. 1987 annual report of the American Association of Poison Control Centers National Data Collection System. Am J Emerg Med 1988;6:479–515.
2. Lettieri DJ, Backenheimer MS. Methodological considerations for a model reporting system of drug deaths. In: Josephson E, Carroll EE, eds. Drug use: epidemiological and sociological approaches. Washington, DC: Hemisphere Publishing, 1974.
3. National Institute on Drug Abuse. Semiannual report: trend data through July–December 1987 — data from the Drug Abuse Warning Network (DAWN). Rockville, Maryland: US Department of Health and Human Services, Public Health Service, 1988. (Series G, no. 21).

[†]The ICD-9 code for unintentional poisoning by drug combinations is E858.8.

4. National Institute on Drug Abuse. Annual data 1987: data from the Drug Abuse Warning Network (DAWN). Rockville, Maryland: US Department of Health and Human Services, Public Health Service, 1988. (Series I, no. 7).
5. Battjes RJ, Jones CL. Implications of etiological research for preventive interventions and future research. In: Jones CL, Battjes RJ, eds. Etiology of drug abuse: implications for prevention. Rockville, Maryland: US Department of Health and Human Services, Public Health Service, 1985; DHHS publication no. (ADM)85-1335. (National Institute on Drug Abuse research monograph no. 56).

Unintentional Ingestions of Prescription Drugs in Children Under Five Years Old

The death rate from poisoning among children younger than 5 years of age has declined by 70% since enactment of the Poison Prevention Packaging Act of 1970. An estimated 86,000 poisonings were prevented between 1974 and 1981. However, the potential for poisoning remains significant. Public education and aware- ness efforts should be targeted at persons who have frequent contact with children, including those who may not live in a household where children reside (e.g., grandparents).

—MMWR Vol. 36/No. 9, March 13, 1987, pp. 124–6, 131–2

Unintentional Ingestions of Prescription Drugs in Children Under Five Years Old

In 1985, the American Association of Poison Control Centers (AAPCC) received more than 60,000 reports of unintentional prescription drug ingestions involving children under the age of five (Consumer Product Safety Commission [CPSC], unpublished data). In addressing this problem, the CPSC initiated a study of the circumstances surrounding oral prescription drug ingestions by children under 5 years of age and of the efficacy of the closures used on the containers involved.

A non-random sample of oral prescription drug ingestions by children was obtained from reports received from February to May 1986 by nine poison control centers representing each of the U.S. Census regions*. Incidents were eligible for the study if the ingestion had been unintentional and had involved a child under 5 years of age. Incidents were excluded if they involved dosing errors or ingestion of veterinary drugs, non-oral prescription drugs, or over-the-counter medications, even if dispensed by prescription. Each center completed 225 investigations. The sample group represented 90% of the eligible reports for the time period.

Trained interviewers administered a telephone questionnaire to parents or other adults present when the ingestion took place. The data collected included 1) the age and sex of the child, 2) the demographics of the child's household, 3) the type of container, 4) who the medicine belonged to and how that person was related to the child, 5) where the child found the medicine, and 6) where the child was when the medicine was consumed. The respondents were also asked to mail the containers to the CPSC so the closures could be examined. Exposures to 1,982 drugs involving 2,015 children met the study criteria.

Seventy-six percent of the ingestions involved children from 1½ to 3½ years of age; 9% were < 1 year or > 4 years old (Table 2). Fifty-six percent of the children were male. The ingested drugs were more frequently owned by female, non-sibling relatives (mother, grandmother, great grandmother, aunt, or cousin) (44%) than by male, non-sibling relatives (12%). Grandparents' medications accounted for a substantial number of episodes (17%).

TABLE 2. Age and sex of children < 5 years of age involved in unintentional ingestions of oral prescription drugs, Consumer Product Safety Commission study, 1986

| Age | Sex | | Total | Percent |
	Males	Females		
< 6 months	1	3	4	0
6 months- < 1 year	19	16	35	2
1 year- < 1½ years	80	71	151	7
1½ years- < 2 years	199	167	366	18
2 years- < 2½ years	282	221	503	25
2½ years- < 3 years	197	157	354	18
3 years- < 3½ years	190	113	303	15
3½ years- < 4 years	84	73	157	8
4 years- < 4½ years	51	38	89	4
4½ years- < 5 years	30	23	53	3
Total	1,133	882	2,015	100

---

*Shreveport, Louisiana; Detroit, Michigan; Pittsburgh, Pennsylvania; Louisville, Kentucky; Minneapolis, Minnesota; District of Columbia; San Diego, California; Boston, Massachusetts; and Salt Lake City, Utah.

Of the 382 containers CPSC received for testing, 80% were child-resistant (Table 3). During follow-up telephone interviews, respondents who had not sent in the containers involved were asked to examine them; 76% of these had child-resistant closures. Sixty-seven percent of respondents who had to base their descriptions on recollection alone reported that the containers had child-resistant closures. Tests proved that 200 (65%) of the 306 child-resistant containers received were ineffective.

TABLE 3. Results of tests of 306 child-resistant containers involved in unintentional ingestions of oral prescription drugs, Consumer Product Safety Commission study, 1986

Type of closure	Number received	Not effective/functional (Percent)
Continuous-thread	229	69
Lug	73	52
Snap	4	75

Two types of child-resistant containers were commonly used. Two hundred and twenty-nine containers used for liquid medications had continuous-thread closures. Sixty-nine percent of these were ineffective; 87% of these failures were associated with a buildup of liquid residue on the threads. Wear of the closure mechanism had caused failure in 52% of the 73 lug-type containers[†].

In 65% of the cases, the medication was in the original container when the ingestion occurred. Problems not related to failure of the child-resistant closure included 1) not resecuring the closure in a child-resistant manner (18% of the incidents), 2) not keeping medicines in any container (i.e., loose), and 3) keeping medicine in some container other than the original (25%). Eighty-two of the ingestions took place in the child's home, and 14%, in a relative's home. The four categories of drugs most frequently ingested were antimicrobials (23.4%), birth control pills and hormones (14.9%), analgesics (9.6%), and cardiovascular drugs (9.2%). The four areas in the home where the ingested medicines were most frequently stored were kitchens (48%), bedrooms (24%), living rooms (10%), and bathrooms (8%).

Reported by American Assn of Poison Control Centers; Div of Poison Prevention and Scientific Coordination, Directorate of Health Sciences, U.S. Consumer Product Safety Commission; Div of Injury Epidemiology and Control, Center for Environmental Health, CDC.

Editorial Note: The week of March 15-21, 1987, is designated National Poison Prevention Week (NPPW) by the Poison Prevention Week Council. NPPW was established by federal legislation and has been observed since 1962 (1). The death rate from poisoning in children under five has steadily declined since the enactment of the Poison Prevention Packaging Act (PPPA) of 1970. Since then, deaths from poisoning by solids and liquids (E850-E866[§]), the group of substances most affected by the PPPA, have declined by 70%. An 8-year analysis of the impact of the PPPA estimated that 86,000 ingestions of poisons were prevented between 1974 and 1981 (2). The potential for poisoning remains significant, however; in 1985,

[†]The majority of the containers received by CPSC were screw-type closures operated by "push and turn" or similar action.

[§]Ninth revision, International Classification of Diseases. The group of external causes E850-E866 excludes gases distributed by pipeline, other utility gases and carbon monoxide, and other gases and vapors since it is not likely that poisoning by these substances would be prevented by the PPPA.

AAPCC centers received more than 500,000 reports of exposures of children under 5 years old to potential poisons (CPSC, unpublished data). In 1983, there were 55 deaths from ingested poisons, 39 of which were from poisoning by drugs, medicinals, and biologicals (E850-E858) (National Center for Health Statistics, unpublished data) (*1*). The age-specific death rate for external causes (E850-E858) in this age group was 0.22/100,000 in 1983 (National Center for Health Statistics, unpublished data) (*3*).

The results of the AAPCC study should be interpreted cautiously since the data were taken from a sample that may not be representative of the entire population under 5 years of age and at risk for poisoning. Furthermore, the purpose of the study was only to determine factors associated with unintended ingestion of oral prescription drugs. In addition, seasonal variation could introduce bias since the data were collected only from February to May.

The findings show that multiple factors contribute to the risk of unintentional ingestion of prescription medications. These include the inability of young children to recognize potential hazards, their tendency to explore the world and to put things in their mouths, and the availability of medicine in the kitchen and bedrooms. Other factors include ineffective child-resistant closures, closures that do not continue to function as designed, and the misuse of these closures.

Public education and awareness efforts should be targeted at persons who have frequent contact with children, including those who may not live in a household where children reside (e.g., grandparents). Unless there are specific reasons to avoid child-resistant containers, consumers who have contact with children should insist on child-resistant packaging regardless of whether they have small children in their own household. Child-resistant containers should always be capped tightly and should never be either modified to eliminate the safety feature or substituted with a non-child-resistant container. Medications should never be kept where children have ready access to them and especially should never be kept in the kitchen or bedrooms.

This study demonstrates the need to use National Poison Prevention Week to make pharmacists, physicians, manufacturers, and the public aware of the importance of the PPPA requirements. While the present technology for child-resistant packaging may provide incomplete protection from prescription drug poisoning, the use of child-resistant packaging should be strongly encouraged whenever possible. Development of improved child-resistant closures with increased reliability should be a priority for the safety-packaging industry. CPSC has made poison prevention a priority project for 1987.

References
1. CDC. National poison prevention week: 25th anniversary observance. MMWR 1986:35;149-52.
2. National Safety Council. Accidental deaths from poisoning. Accident Facts 1982:82-3.
3. Bureau of the Census. Resident population in thousands by age, sex, and race. Washington, DC: U.S. Department of Commerce, Bureau of the Census, 1984. (Table 2; series P-25; no. 949).

Carbon Monoxide Poisoning Associated with a Propane-Powered Floor Burnisher — Vermont, 1992

Deaths resulting from carbon monoxide (CO) poisoning are more common in winter months. Prevention efforts should be aimed at persons who live in homes with old heating systems, gas-powered space heaters, or wood stoves.

—MMWR Vol. 42/No. 37, September 24, 1993, pp. 726–8

Carbon Monoxide Poisoning Associated with a Propane-Powered Floor Burnisher — Vermont, 1992

On July 28, 1992, two employees of a pharmacy in Vermont fainted within four hours after arriving for work; at a local hospital emergency department, carbon monoxide (CO) poisoning was diagnosed based on elevated carboxyhemoglobin (HbCO) levels. The pharmacy was evacuated, and the remaining eight employees were transported to the hospital for evaluation. Further investigation by the Vermont Department of Health (VDH) revealed that, on July 24, one of the employees had fainted, but CO poisoning was not suspected, and vasovagal syncope was diagnosed. This report summarizes the investigation of these cases by VDH.

A case of CO poisoning was defined as an arterial HbCO ≥2% (for nonsmokers) or ≥9% (for smokers) (1) in an employee who worked at the pharmacy on July 28. Based on analysis of arterial blood samples, nine of the 10 employees met the case definition; six were women. The mean age was 26.8 years (range: 17–42 years). Reported symptoms included headache (nine patients), lightheadedness (seven), tunnel vision (five), nausea/vomiting (four), syncope (two), difficulty breathing (two), chest pain (two), and decreased hearing (one). Serum samples were taken from six case-patients within 1½ hours of exposure and from the other three case-patients within 3 hours of exposure. Mean HbCO was 16.6% (range: 6.7%–25.3%). Three patients received hyperbaric oxygen therapy: one had psychometric test abnormalities, and two had syncope without psychometric testing. All nine patients recovered.

On both July 24 and July 28, the store's floors had been cleaned with a liquid propane-powered floor burnisher by a subcontractor to a cleaning service company. The floor burnisher was independently owned and operated. On both days, the subcontractor had cleaned and polished the pharmacy floors before employees arrived. No cases of illness consistent with CO poisoning were reported among cleaning service employees.

The Division of Occupational and Radiological Health, VDH, impounded the burnisher and tested its emissions 2 days after the incident. Readings obtained outdoors from the burnisher's exhaust pipe reached 2000 parts per million (ppm) CO after less than 1 minute of measurement, 3000 ppm while idling, and 50,000 ppm at full throttle. All other possible sources of CO (i.e., heating and air-conditioning system, water-heater system, and truck traffic outside the store) were excluded as causes of the exposure.

HbCO levels among case-patients were used to estimate CO concentration in the work environment by the Coburn equation (2); this approach estimated that, on the morning of exposure, the CO concentration in the pharmacy was 507–1127 ppm. The Occupational Safety and Health Administration (OSHA) standard for CO is 50 ppm averaged over an 8-hour work shift and a ceiling level of 200 ppm, not to be exceeded at any time. The store's ventilation system used 100% recirculated air.

As a result of this investigation, the pharmacy and the cleaning contractor and subcontractor were fined. VDH recommended that liquid propane-powered burnishers be replaced with electric-powered burnishers and that CO alarms be installed if use of liquid propane-powered machines continued.

Reported by: K Uraneck, MD, Southwestern Vermont Medical Center, Bennington; R McCandless, MPH, S Meyer, R Houseknecht, PhD, L Paulozzi, MD, State Epidemiologist, Vermont Dept of Health. Div of Field Epidemiology, Epidemiology Program Office, CDC.

Editorial Note: Unintentional exposure to CO is a major environmental hazard in the United States (*3,4*): each year, approximately 10,000 persons seek medical attention because of CO intoxication (*5*). Unintentional deaths attributable to CO poisoning result primarily from combustion of gasoline in motor vehicles, coal for heating or cooking, kerosene, and wood (*3,6*). In contrast to these fuels, propane—the source of fuel involved in this report—normally undergoes complete combustion in the presence of sufficient oxygen, producing nontoxic CO_2 and water vapor (*7*); only when the oxygen supply at the point of combustion is inadequate does combustion of propane produce CO.

Symptoms of mild CO poisoning are nonspecific, and affected persons may not seek medical care. Because the cleaning service employees involved in the episode described in this report were exposed to elevated CO levels for limited periods (i.e., less than 1 hour), they may not have suffered ill effects of exposure. Pharmacy employees likely were exposed to peak CO levels on arrival to work and to elevated levels throughout the day.

The floor burnisher involved in this incident was factory-labeled with a warning to "shut off the engine if headache occurs and check emissions." OSHA permissible exposure levels regulate indoor air quality but do not require that such machines meet emission standards or receive routine maintenance. The most likely cause of CO poisoning in this case was failure to maintain or routinely service the burnisher. In addition, inadequate ventilation may have contributed to elevated concentrations of CO in the work environment. Episodes of CO poisoning, such as that described in this report, can be prevented by using only electric burnishers indoors, maintaining and routinely servicing fuel-burning burnishers, ensuring proper ventilation of the workplace, and educating persons regarding the signs and symptoms of CO poisoning.

Deaths resulting from CO poisoning are more common in winter months (*3*). Prevention efforts should be aimed at persons who live in homes with old heating systems, gas-powered space heaters, or wood stoves. Proper use and maintenance of such home-heating systems and cleaning of obstructed chimneys can prevent CO poisoning in the home.

References
1. CDC. Unintentional deaths from carbon monoxide poisoning—Michigan, 1987–1989. MMWR 1992;41:881–3,889.
2. Coburn RF, Forster RE, Kane PB. Considerations of the physiology and variables that determine the blood carboxyhemoglobin concentration in man. J Clin Invest 1965;41:1899–910.
3. Cobb N, Etzel RA. Unintentional carbon monoxide-related deaths in the United States, 1979–1988. JAMA 1991;266:659–63.
4. CDC. Unintentional carbon monoxide poisoning following a winter storm—Washington, January 1993. MMWR 1993;42:109–11.
5. Schaplowsky AF, Oglesbay FB, Morrison JH, Gallagher RE, Berman W. Carbon monoxide contamination of the living environment: a national survey of home air and children's blood. Journal of Environmental Health 1974;36:569–73.
6. Baron RC, Backer RC, Sopher IM. Fatal unintended carbon monoxide poisoning in West Virginia from nonvehicular sources. Am J Public Health 1989;79:1656–8.
7. American Gas Association. Fundamentals of gas combustion. Arlington, Virginia: American Gas Association, 1973; catalog no. XH0373.

Lay Involvement in Health and Other Research

Alan Earl-Slater

RADCLIFFE MEDICAL PRESS

Radcliffe Medical Press Ltd
18 Marcham Road
Abingdon
Oxon OX14 1AA
United Kingdom

www.radcliffe-oxford.com
The Radcliffe Medical Press electronic catalogue and online ordering facility.
Direct sales to anywhere in the world.

_____

British Library Cataloguing in Publication Data

A catalogue record for this book is available from the British Library.

ISBN 1 85775 847 1

Typeset by Advance Typesetting Ltd, Oxford
Printed and bound by TJ International Ltd, Padstow, Cornwall